CHICAGO PUBLIC LIBRARY

R00977 58814

CHICAGO PUBLIC LIBRARY

D0908608

OGY

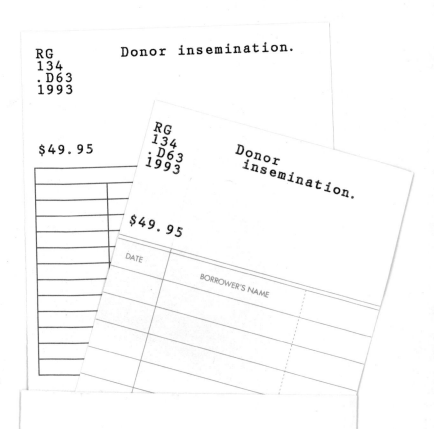

RG
134
.D63
1993

Donor insemination.

$49.95

RG
134
.D63
1993

Donor
insemination.

$49.95

DATE	BORROWER'S NAME	

DISCARD

BAKER & TAYLOR BOOKS

This volume provides clear guidelines on the advantages, disadvantages and limitations of the use of donor insemination to treat infertility. The team of authors, drawn from a wide range of disciplines, covers all aspects of implementing and organizing a successful donor insemination programme. The volume includes practical information on recruitment, screening and selection of suitable donors; counselling of patients and donors; clinical, scientific and laboratory aspects, including fertility assessment, ovulation timing and cryopreservation. The volume concludes with information on organization of sperm banks, the use of computerization and ethical and legal aspects.

The volume is designed to assist all those involved in the treatment of infertility – including andrologists and clinicians in the fields of reproductive medicine and obstetrics and gynaecology.

DONOR INSEMINATION

DONOR INSEMINATION

C. L. R. BARRATT and I. D. COOKE

University Department of Obstetrics and Gynaecology,
Jessop Hospital for Women, Sheffield, UK

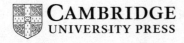

CAMBRIDGE
UNIVERSITY PRESS

Published by the Press Syndicate of the University of Cambridge
The Pitt Building, Trumpington Street, Cambridge CB2 1RP
40 West 20th Street, New York, NY 10011-4211, USA
10 Stamford Road, Oakleigh, Melbourne 3166, Australia

© Cambridge University Press 1993

First published 1993

Printed in Great Britain at the University Press, Cambridge

A catalogue record for this book is available from the British Library

Library of Congress cataloguing in publication data
Donor insemination/[editors] C. L. R. Barratt and I. D. Cooke.
    p.   cm.
  Includes index.
  ISBN 0-521-40433-9
  1. Artificial insemination, Human.   I. Barratt, C. L. R.
II. Cooke, I. D. (Ian Douglas)
RG134.D63   1993
618.1'78—dc20 92-32194 CIP

ISBN 0 521 40433 9   hardback

ROO977 58814

Contents

Contributors

R. J. Aitken
MRC Reproductive Biology Unit, Centre for Reproductive Biology, 37 Chalmers Street, Edinburgh EH3 9EW, UK

C. L. R. Barratt
University Department of Obstetrics & Gynaecology, Jessop Hospital for Women, Sheffield S3 7RE, UK

G. M. Centola
Department of Obstetrics & Gynaecology, Box 668, University of Rochester Medical Centre, 601 Elmwood Avenue, Rochester, New York 14642, USA

M. Chauhan
Department of Obstetrics & Gynaecology, Newcastle General Hospital, Westgate Road, Newcastle upon Tyne, UK

I. D. Cooke
University Department of Obstetrics & Gynaecology, Jessop Hospital for Women, Sheffield S3 7RE, UK

S. Cooke
University Department of Obstetrics & Gynaecology, Jessop Hospital for Women, Sheffield S3 7RE, UK

E. Z. Drobnis
Zoology Department, University of California, Davis, California 95616, USA

B. A. Keel
The Center for Reproductive Medicine, The Women's Research Institute, Department of Obstetrics & Gynaecology, HCA/Wesley Medical Center,

University of Kansas School of Medicine-Wichita, 2903 E. Central, Wichita, KS 67214, USA

G. T. Kovacs
Infertility Medical Centre, Epworth Hospital, 61 Erin Street, Richmond, Melbourne, Victoria 3121, Australia

E. J. Lamb
Department of Obstetrics & Gynaecology, Stamford University School of Medicine, Stamford, California, USA

J. Lansac
CECOS du Centre-Ouest, CHR Bretonneau, bd Tonnèle, 37044, Tours, France

H. Leach
University Department of Obstetrics & Gynaecology, Jessop Hospital for Women, Sheffield S3 7RE, UK

E. A. Lenton
University Department of Obstetrics & Gynaecology, Jessop Hospital for Women, Sheffield S3 7RE, UK

D. Le Lannou
CECOS de l'Ouest, CHR Hotel-Dieu, rue de la Cochardière, 35000, Rennes, France

I. McLeod
University Department of Obstetrics & Gynaecology, Jessop Hospital for Women, Sheffield S3 7RE, UK

J. C. Osborn
Centre for Early Human Development, Monash University, Monash Medical Centre, 246 Clayton Road, Clayton, Melbourne, Victoria 3188, Australia

J. Overstreet
Department of Obstetrics & Gynaecology School of Medicine, University of California, Davis, California 95616, USA

D. W. Richardson
MRC Reproductive Biology Unit, 37 Chalmers Street, Edinburgh EH3 9EW, UK

R. Snowden
Department of Population Studies, University of Exeter, UK

B. W. Webster
The Center for Reproductive Medicine, The Women's Research Institute,
Department of Obstetrics & Gynaecology, HCA/Wesley Medical Center,
University of Kansas School of Medicine-Wichita, 2903 E. Central,
Wichita, KS 67214, USA

C. A. Yates
Infertility Medical Centre, Epworth Hospital, 61 Erin Street, Richmond,
Melbourne, Victoria 3121, Australia

1

Introduction

I. D. COOKE

Donor insemination is the most widespread and successful form of assisted reproduction. The American Fertility Society and the American Association of Tissue Banks reported that there were over 30 000 births as a result of donor insemination in the United States in 1987, whereas, even in 1990, the number of births by GIFT and IVF combined in the USA was only just over 3000.

Recently there appears to have been a revival of interest in donor insemination (DI). This is likely to be due to several factors.

1. Frozen semen has been used exclusively to reduce the transmission of HIV to a recipient. Frozen semen, many believe, is less effective than fresh semen, and therefore considerable effort has been made to improve success rates including developing more successful techniques of cryopreservation.
2. The legislation/recommendations of the Code of Practice associated with DI, particularly in the United Kingdom, where centres are licensed and inspected by the Human Fertilization and Embryology Authority have dramatically changed the practices of DI.
3. The generally increased interest and experience in other reproductive technology, e.g. GIFT, IVF and micromanipulation have led to a re-evaluation of the role and success of DI and to an integration of various techniques to achieve conception.

However, despite the widespread use of DI, and its success in the treatment of male infertility, research is minimal compared to those of other techniques. There is clearly a paucity of specific controlled trials which are necessary to answer important biological questions, e.g. the number of inseminations necessary for optimum fecundability.

Throughout the book, particular points have been emphasized: (1) some advances have been made, e.g. techniques to accurately detect ovulation; methods to examine the fertilizing capacity of donor semen. Such advances are highlighted and discussed. It is hoped that such information will assist with the clinical management of the patients by emphasizing factors which affect DI success rates. (2) In donor insemination, many factors governing the success of the reproductive system can be controlled. Thus donor insemination can serve as an excellent system for research. Provided that donors with high fertilizing capacity are used consistently, other factors affecting success can be studied, e.g. subtle defects in the reproductive system. There appear to be very few scientists or clinicians who make use of this highly controlled system. It is hoped that the information in this book will encourage investigators to perform studies which add to understanding and treatment capabilities.

2

Donor recruitment, selection and screening

C. L. R. BARRATT

One of the major problems for donor insemination centres is the recruitment of suitable donors who are healthy, free from transmissible genetic disorders, sexually transmitted diseases, including acquired immune deficiency syndrome, and have semen with high fertilizing potential (Barratt, Chauhan & Cooke, 1990).

Until recently, there has been a paucity of information on the current practices for the screening of semen donors. This was highlighted in a survey of the donor insemination clinics registered with the Royal College of Obstetricians and Gynaecologists in the United Kingdom. It was concluded that there was no systematic comprehensive approach by donor insemination clinics to prevent the spread of common sexually transmissible pathogens to recipients (Barratt *et al.*, 1989). A survey in the United States, completed by the office of Technology and Assessment, presented disturbing evidence that there was a lack of a structured rational approach to the screening of semen donors (OTA, 1988). Surprisingly, a large percentage of physicians were unaware of the specific professional guidelines for the screening of semen donors, i.e. the American Fertility Society guidelines (AFS 1986), although many of the sperm banks adhered to such regulations.

Selection of donors

In the United Kingdom, students constitute the major demographic group of donors (75%), married men with children being specifically recruited in only 25% of DI centres (Barratt *et al.*, 1989). All donors are recruited mainly by word of mouth but also by specific advertisements in the University and Polytechnic Press; the donors are often paid a fee which generally covers travelling expenses. One of the major advantages

3

of recruiting student donors is that enough donors can be recruited to satisfy the needs of the individual clinics. However, the major disadvantage is that they are often not of proven fertility and, in the United Kingdom, the HFEA strongly recommend that semen donors should now be recruited from men who already have children and are in a stable relationship (HFEA, 1991). Another problem with recruiting student donors is that they are young (18–24 years) and sexually active. Therefore, the incidence of sexually transmitted disease is higher than what one would expect in men with children in a stable relationship, e.g. urethral pathogens have been detected in one-third of potential semen donors (Monteiro *et al.*, 1987). In France, recruitment of donors is confined to men from couples with one or more children where the donation is anonymous and there is no fee paid. As a result of the guidelines for DI advocated by the HFEA it is likely that the recruitment profile of donors will change dramatically as proven fertile men are recruited and are in a stable relationship (HFEA, 1991). These men can be recruited from vasectomy clinics, from friends of infertile couples or may be recruited by advertising locally or nationally. Attempts have been made to recruit men through antenatal classes but level of recruitment is very low (approximately 1%) and efforts are now being renewed to recruit men from vasectomy clinics and from advertisements in the local and national press. In order to recruit a suitable number of donors, a constant campaign needs to be vigorously maintained.

Screening donors for sexually transmitted disease

The risk of transmission of pathogens to recipients of donor insemination was highlighted by Stewart in 1985 (Stewart *et al.*, 1985) when they documented the transmission of HIV to four out of eight recipients of cryopreserved semen from a donor without symptoms. This acount stimulated several reviews of mainly anecdotal reports of the transmission of genital pathogens including Ureaplasma, HIV and Neisseria to recipients of donor semen (Mascola & Guinan 1986; Greenblatt *et al.*, 1986). Two more recent reports of the transmission of cytomegalovirus (CMV) (Demmler *et al.*, 1986) and Herpes simplex virus type 2 (Moore *et al.*, 1989) have again highlighted the risks associated with donor insemination and the problems of screening donors. The transmission of Herpes simplex virus type 2 has been confirmed by finding identical restriction enzyme patterns in a semen recipient and the donor (Moore *et al.*, 1989). The virus was transmitted to only one or two recipients of fresh semen from a donor who was without symptoms. This report raises an important issue in screening donors as over two-thirds of the people who are positive for Herpes simplex virus type 2 have no history of genital lesions (Barratt & Cooke, 1989). These data suggest that transmission of the virus could not be eliminated by making a detailed history and a physical examination. Cytomegalovirus (CMV) has been documented to be transferred by fresh semen to a recipient (Demmler *et al.*, 1986). Molecular analysis of the CMV from virus isolated from the male and the female partner showed strain homology and provided conclusive evidence that the female contracted the CMV from her stable partner. Hammitt and colleagues showed that CMV could be recovered from the semen of one of four donors seropositive for cytomegalovirus even after the semen had been frozen for up to 9 months (Hammitt, Aschenbrenner & Williamson, 1988). This finding has important implications. First, it shows that freezing does not inactivate the virus (HIV: Stewart *et al.*, 1985; Herpes simplex virus: Sherman & Menna, 1986 also survive freezing), and secondly it provides further support for the viewpoint that all semen donor should be seronegative for cytomegalovirus (AFS, 1990).

The true incidence of the transmission of these and other pathogens in donor insemination needs to be determined as there have been no large prospective microbiological studies. This information is clearly necessary to evaluate the risks to the recipients of DI. The establishment of multicentre studies to evaluate the presence of sexually transmitted disease in potential donors and their complication in recipients has been encouraged (Barratt *et al.*, 1989), but we still await the results from these studies (Barratt & Cooke, 1989). We also need to know the most effective method of screening potential donors. This question is very much open to debate (see Barratt *et al.*, 1989; Barratt & Cooke, 1989; 1990). Many groups have formulated guidelines for screening semen donors (see above). These guidelines show that there is a consensus in some matters, e.g. the exclusive use of frozen semen to allow the serum of the donor to be tested and cleared for HIV antibodies, the use of urethral swabs to detect sexually transmitted diseases, and an adequate physical examination and history taking. The use of such guidelines will greatly restrict the transmission of pathogens to recipients. Yet, as recently as 1988, there was no systematic approach by donor insemination clinics in the United Kingdom to prevent the spread of common sexually transmitted pathogens to the recipients (Barratt *et al.*, 1989), e.g. only 9% of clinics carried out urethral tests suggested as mandatory 15 months earlier by the American Fertility Society (AFS, 1986). Even in the United States, despite specific guidelines, a national survey in 1987 also indicated a lack of a structured approach (OTA, 1988). Over half of the physicians who performed donor insemination were unaware of professional guidelines for recruiting semen donors. In response to this, the American Fertility Society has recently updated its guidelines on the use of semen for donor insemination (AFS, 1990). They conclude that careful screening of the potential donors, together with routine surveillance of their health, are important methods of reducing the risks of infection, and that it is of primary importance to establish a good rapport with potential donors so that an in-depth knowledge of the health status is obtained. The American Fertility Society suggests completing a detailed history of the potential donors only after several semen samples have been examined and considered suitable. If the donor is suitable, e.g. no evidence of sexually transmitted disease in the last 6 months, a blood sample should be taken and screened for hepatitis, HIV, syphilis and CMV antibodies, although screening for the latter is contentious (see Chauhan *et al.*, 1989). A physical examination is then performed which includes urethral tests for *Neisseria* and *Chlamydia*, swabs for *Mycoplasma hominis* and *Trichomonas vaginalis* are optional, as is detection of white blood cells. The physical examination includes making certain that there is no urethral discharge, genital warts or genital ulcers.

A similar rationalized and objective protocol has been developed for the screening of potential donors (see Table 2.1) based on previous experiences (see Chauhan *et al.*, 1988).

In contrast to the AFS, it is recommended that the first stage of recruitment should be the completion of a questionnaire which serves to exclude donors considered to be unsuitable (usually 15% to 25% in the author's clinic). Subsequently, a semen sample is produced and, if this is acceptable, the potential donors are given a physical examination, urethral tests and appropriate tests for HIV, hepatitis, VDRL and CMV. This procedure reduces the financial burden, as a large number of potential donors are rejected because of unsuitable semen characteristics (−60%). Recommendations for screening prospective semen donors to exclude sexually transmitted infections are outlined in Table 2.1. The donors are then re-screened to exclude them if there are any symptomatic signs for STD, genital warts, genital herpes, genital ulcers and urethral discharge every 6 months at a minimum. Re-screening of donors for all the above also takes place at the time of completion of donations. As mainly students are recruited, it would be impractical to exclude donors who have a new sexual partner during their period of donation, as

Table 2.1. *Recommendations for prospective screening of semen donors in the UK to exclude sexually transmitted infections*

Initial screening
1. Precounselling
   Exclude all men in high-risk groups for HIV
2. History
   Current genital symptoms
   Previous history of STD
   Sexual history (number of sexual partners in previous 6 months)
3. Genital examination
   Genital ulcer disease
   Genital warts
   Urethral discharge
4. Urethral tests (men should hold their urine for 4 h preceding these tests
   Gram-stained smear
   Neisseria gonorrhoeae
   Chlamydia trachomatis
   Ureaplasma urealyticum
   Mycoplasma hominis
   Trichomonas vaginalis
5. Serological tests
   Human immunodeficiency virus antibody
   Treponema pallidum (VDRL, TPHA)
   Cytomegalovirus antibody
   Hepatitis B virus (HbsAg, antiHbc)
6. Exclude all men who have a history or evidence of any viral STD (including hepatitis B virus); treat those men who have STD; arrange follow-up and contact tracing; reconsider as donors those men who have microbiologically cured bacterial STD and a stable sexual relationship
7. Obtain adequate specimens of semen
8. Use CMV-seronegative men as universal donors; CMV-seropositive donors should donate to CMV-seropositive recipients only

Follow-up of regular donors
   Re-screen donors every 6 months and at the last donation for points 2, 3, 4, 5 as a relevant history should be sought at each donation

recommended by the AFS (AFS, 1990). It is, however, stressed to all our donors that they use a condom during that period of donation, and, for their own protection and safety, that they restrict the number of partners to an absolute minimum.

One of the interesting and contentious issues in the recruitment of donors has been the exclusion criteria used for STD. In a survey of the United Kingdom clinics, very few centres ask for the details of genital tract disease or perform a genital examination (Barratt *et al.*, 1989). Information obtained in this way is very useful in assessing the current and future risk of STD, and in facilitating the diagnosis of active genital infections and conditions such as HIV infection for which there are currently no routine laboratory tests. It was found that most centres exclude men if they have a previous history of STD infections such as gonorrhoea, non-gonococcal urethritis and syphilis. Many clinics fail to ask specifically about the history of a viral infection. It is recommended that only men who have a history of viral STD including hepatitis virus be excluded (see Table 2.1). Men with a history of urethritis are accepted if shown to be negative at the time of screening.

The American Fertility Society recommends that only CMV seronegative donors be used (AFS, 1990). This is a difficult policy to implement as up to 40% of semen donors have antibodies to CMV (Chauhan *et al.*, 1989). It is feasible to match CMV-negative recipients to CMV-negative donors. However, there are problems in the exclusive use of CMV negative donors; for example, this would compound the difficulty in recruiting sufficient numbers of good quality donors. Many questions about CMV remain unanswered, e.g. transmission of the different viral strains, reactivation of the latent virus, effects of cryopreservation on the various viral strains and secretion rates of the virus into semen. Future research into these areas is clearly necessary so that informed decisions about the use of CMV positive donors can be made. In the meantime the use of CMV negative donors is recommended whenever possible but always on CMV negative recipients. In the author's clinic, CMV positive donors are only matched with CMV positive recipients. Attempts have recently been made to isolate and culture CMV from seropositive donors. To date, over 400 semen samples have been screened from ten seropositive donors and there has been failure to isolate the CMV virus. However, the secretion into semen is known to be periodic, highlighting the question 'should we screen all donor semen samples for CMV?'.

The transmission of HIV by donor insemination merits special attention. To reduce the risk of transmission of the virus, there is now universal acceptance for the exclusive use of frozen semen in donor insemination clinics. This has recently been stressed by the American Fertility Society, which recommends the exclusive use of frozen semen that has been quarantined for 6 months and the donor re-tested and found to be seronegative for HIV before the specimen is released (AFS, 1990). It is therefore absolutely necessary for a good rapport to be established with the donors so that a semen sample can be obtained 180 days after the last semen donation. The Department of Health in the United Kingdom still recommend a 3-month period, and there has been controversy over this in the literature. It is interesting in this context to note that the modelling of cases of HIV infection with known exposure in published reports gave a median of 2.4 months from exposure to antibody detection, and 95% of the cases would be expected to seroconvert within 5.8 months. HIV infection for longer than 6 months without detectable antibody was uncommon (Horsburgh *et al.*, 1989). Based on this report, it would be clinically negligent to use less than a 6-month quarantine period. As this field is rapidly expanding, clinicians and scientists should be constantly aware of future developments that may have a dramatic impact on donor insemination, e.g. the time from exposure to the virus and antibody production and the availability of a routine test to detect the antigen in semen.

Genetic screening for gamete donors

Several authors have stressed that donor screening for genetic diseases has, in the past, been grossly inadequate, e.g. in the OTA survey in 1987 some physicians stated that they would reject healthy donors with a family history of sex-linked disorders that are not transmittable unless the donor himself has the condition (OTA, 1988). There is therefore a need to improve the genetic screening of potential donors. The American Fertility Society has recently published an excellent review of this screening providing detailed examples (AFS, 1990). Their screening is usually obtained from a detailed history of the donor which can either can be carried out very early in the programme as recommended by Schroeder-Jenkins (Schroeder-Jenkins & Rothman, 1989) or after the production of semen samples as recommended by the American Fertility Society (AFS, 1990) and by Chauhan *et al.*, 1988. The screening should be performed by a qualified medical person who is aware of the minimal genetic screening for donors. It is important to remember that the level of competence at questioning is extremely important in obtaining the genetic screening by history, e.g. Timmons and colleagues, using exten- sive data, interview and collection systems found that 5.4% of 149 donors had self-assessed genetic disorders; elsewhere extensive investigation revealed that 29.5% had conditions within the family which warranted further investigation, a 5.5 fold discrepancy (Timmons *et al.*, 1981). The author's own programme is based on a thorough checklist of specific conditions plus a medical interview. This results in a rejection rate of approximately only 1%. There is always close consultation with our local genetic colleagues on any doubtful issues to obtain a balanced approach and this close co-operation is recommended.

Conclusions

With the increasing difficulty and the strict guidelines for recruiting semen donors, many clinics will be unable to recruit sufficient numbers of donors and therefore have to obtain semen from other centres. With the situation likely to get worse, for example, and the movement in the United Kingdom towards the recruitment of fertile men, we would advocate the setting up of regional centres to recruit donors; all such donors could have their semen specifically tested for fertilizing potential using sophisticated sperm function testing (see Aitken, Chapter 5). A well thought-out, structured, rationalized protocol for the investigation of semen donors is advocated and it is suggested that, in the United Kingdom, the Royal College of Obstetrics and Gynaecologists or the British Andrology Society should provide such guidelines equivalent to those of the American Fertility Society to help DI centres formulate their policy.

References

American Fertility Society (AFS) (1986). New guidelines for the use of semen for donor insemination. *Fertility and Sterility*, **46**(suppl): 95S.

American Fertility Society (AFS) (1990). New guidelines for the use of semen for donor insemination. *Fertility and Sterility*, **53**, Suppl. 1.

Barratt, C. L. R., Chauhan, M. & Cooke, I. D. (1990). Donor insemination – a look to the future. *Fertility and Sterility,* **54**, 375–87.

Barratt, C. L. R. & Cooke, I. D. (1989). Risks of donor insemination. *British Medical Journal*, **299**, 1178–9.

Barratt, C. L. R. & Cooke, I. D. (1990). Risks of donor insemination. A review. *International Journal of Risk & Safety Medicine*, **1**, 113–15.

Barratt, C. L. R., Monteiro, E. F., Chauhan, M., Cooke, S. & Cooke, I. D. (1989). Screening donors for sexually transmitted disease in donor insemination clinics in the UK. A survey. *British Journal of Obstetrics and Gynaecology*, **96**, 461–6.

Chauhan, M., Barratt, C. L. R., Cooke, S. & Cooke, I. D. (1988). A protocol for the recruitment and screening of semen donors for an artificial insemination by donor programme. *Human Reproduction*, **3**, 873–6.

Chauhan, M., Barratt, C. L. R., Cooke, S. & Cooke, I. D. (1989). Screening for cytomegalovirus antibody in a donor insemination program: difficulties in implementing The American Fertility Society guidelines. *Fertility and Sterility*, **51**, 901–2.

Demmler, G. J., O'Neil, G. W., O'Neil, J. H., Spector, S. A., Brady, M. T. & Yow, M. D. (1986). Transmission of Cytomegalovirus from husband to wife (letter). *Journal of Infectious Diseases*, **154**, 545–6.

Greenblatt, R. M., Handsfield, H. H., Sayers, M. H. & Holmes, K. K. (1986). Screening therapeutic insemination donors for sexually transmitted diseases: overview and recommendations. *Fertility and Sterility*, **46**, 351–64.

Hammitt, D. G., Aschenbrenner, B. S. & Williamson, R. A. (1988). Culture of cytomegalovirus from frozen-thawed semen. *Fertility and Sterility*, **49**, 554–7.

HFEA (1991). Code of practice. Human Fertilisation and Embryology Authority, London.

Horsbergh, C. R. J., Jason, J., Longini, I. M. *et al.* (1989). Duration of human immunodeficiency virus infection before detection of antibody. *Lancet*, 637–40.

Mascola, L. M. & Guinan, M. E. (1986). Screening to reduce transmission of sexually transmitted diseases in semen used for artificial insemination. *New England Journal of Medicine*, 1354–9.

Monteiro, E. F., Spencer, R. C., Kinghorn, G. R., Barratt, C. L. R., Cooke, S. & Cooke, I. D. (1987). Sexually transmitted disease in potential semen donors. *British Medical Journal*, **295**, 418.

Moore, D. E., Ashley, R. L., Zarutskie, P. W., Coombs, R. W. Soules, M. R. & Corey, L. (1989). Transmission of genital herpes by donor insemination. *Journal of the American Medical Association*, **261**, 3441–3.

Office of Technology and Assessment (OTA). (1988). *Congress of the United States: Artificial Insemination: Practice in the United States*. US Government, Washington, p.112.

Schroeder-Jenkins, M. & Rothman, S. A. (1989). Causes of donor rejection in a sperm banking program. *Fertility and Sterility*, **51**, 903–6.

Sherman, J. K. & Menna, J. H. (1986). Brief Communication. Cryosurvival of Herpes simplex virus-2 during cryopreservation of human spermatazoa. *Cryobiology*, **23**, 383–5.

Stewart, G. J., Cunningham, A. L., Driscoll, G. L., Tyler, J. P. P., Barr, J. A. & Gold, J. (1985). Transmission of human T-cell lymphotropic virus type III (HTLV-III) by artificial insemination by donor. *Lancet*, **ii**, 581–4.

Timmons, M. C., Rao, K. W., Sloan, C. S., Kirkman, H. N. & Talbert, L. N. (1981). Genetic screening of donors for artificial insemination. *Fertility and Sterility*, **35**, 451–6.

3

Counselling in donor insemination

S. COOKE

As new treatments offer increasing hope to childless couples, the effects of the new technology have highlighted the value of counselling. Few people would dispute that such couples should have the opportunity to discuss their fertility problem and its implications in a caring and supportive way with well-informed staff.

When the problem is one of male infertility, it has not always been easy to know what kind of help is required, when it should be offered and by whom. Increasingly, it is becoming clear that sympathetic, supportive counselling to help such couples come to terms with the diagnosis is seen by them as a priority. Their feelings of loss and isolation need to be heard and discussed long before they are able to think about treatment, and this aspect is often unrecognized.

This chapter tries to identify the potential problems faced by such couples and how best to help them not only by sympathetic support but also by well-informed discussion. Treatment options are detailed, but the main emphasis is on the choice and long-term effects of donor insemination. Secrecy and openness are considered together with the implications of the recent Human Fertilisation and Embryology Act (UK, 1990). Choice of donor, timing of insemination and success rates are discussed. Donor selection, screening and donor counselling are also examined.

Problems faced by couples; the need for support

From their own experience, many infertile couples feel that the medical profession, with limited time for consultation, cannot be expected to give the best counselling however well intentioned. Because their training teaches them primarily to make a diagnosis and offer treatment, they may fail to recognize the acute emotional trauma experienced by many couples faced for the first time with a fertility problem. It should be remembered that, in a world which assumes that easy procreation is the norm, and the right of those who desire it, infertile couples often see themselves as abnormal, misfits and social outcasts. They may have difficulty understanding how this could have happened to them. How can they tell their families and friends? What will other people think? There are often feelings of isolation, frustration and anger. To be told a much wanted child is not going to arrive can, for many, produce the intensity of a bereavement and a certain amount of grieving has to be worked through. A non-medical counsellor, social worker, psychologist or sympathetic communicator from whatever discipline has a key role to play at this time. However, people's needs vary. Some couples will prefer to work through such an experience by themselves or with an understanding family and friends, and to be forced into prolonged psycho-analytical discussion would be counterproductive. It seems necessary that such supportive counselling should be available and offered to infertile couples before treatment is considered, but should be acknowledged as voluntary.

Infertility is generally considered to be a 'woman's problem'. There is a tendency for men to think of fertility and virility as synonymous, a myth that needs to be dispelled, so it is not surprising that, when the problem is attributed to the man, it may be perceived as a denial of masculinity, and the effect can be devastating. A retrospective investigation of 843 couples attending an infertility clinic over a 10-year period found that both men and women reported greater emotional distress and marital difficulties when the cause of the infertility lay with the man (Connolly, Edelmann & Cooke, 1987).

A great deal depends on how the diagnosis of male infertility is conveyed to the couple, and doctors in such a position should be aware of the consequences of what they say. A study by Berger (1980) found that 11 husbands out of 16 interviewed experienced impotence for 1–4 months after hearing of their infertility. However, this was not the finding of Humphrey & Humphrey (1987) in a group of 100 couples where very few admitted to sexual problems; perhaps the time-gap in the studies reflects an easing of social attitudes. A further study of 120 couples by Berger *et al.* (1986) discusses the anger and guilt felt by the women and their anxiety to protect their husbands. Many women say they wish the problem rested with them!

It is never easy to give bad news. A compassionate and supportive approach, an explanation which puts the problem in perspective, offers of additional counselling and discussion, and details of local and national infertility support groups are a good start. No couple presented with the diagnosis of male infertility should feel abandoned and left to cope alone with their problem as best they can.

To compound the problem, acceptance of male infertility has to incorporate the fact that, for the present, there is little to offer in the way of treatment, although interest in the field is increasing. Coming to terms with the situation may take many months or, in some instances, many years before couples feel ready to look at their options. At that stage, they need time for well-informed discussion and an opportunity to explore alternatives with an emphasis on the implications and possible long-term consequences of any decision.

Options available

Treatment

Unfortunately this will only be appropriate for a few, with very limited guarantee of success.

Previous vasectomy

Vasectomy reversal may be the treatment of choice but the outcome is variable, and results are often expressed as the number with sperm found as opposed to the more relevant subsequent pregnancy rate. Sperm quality may be compromised by the presence of antibodies attached to the sperm only identifiable in a post-reversal ejaculate.

Sperm antibodies

A resurgence of interest in treating sperm antibodies with intermittent low-dose steroids has in one double-blind, cross-over trial produced a cumulative pregnancy rate of 31% at 9 months (Hendry *et al.*, 1990).

Testicular obstruction

Acquired blocks of the cauda epididymis, the vas deferens or the ejaculatory ducts are potentially suitable for surgical correction (Hendry,

1988). Encouragingly, a pregnancy has recently been achieved in Australia using sperm recovered from the caput epididymis (Jequier *et al.*, 1990). In congenital absence of the vas, sperm may be recovered from the rete testis and, by IVF, produce a pregnancy (Silber *et al.*, 1988).

Oligozoospermia

Pregnancies have been described with low sperm densities using IVF. In severe oligozoospermia (<5 million motile sperm/ml) fertilization rates are significantly lower than in those considered normospermic (>12 million motile sperm/ml). Fertilization rates appear to be normal with moderate oligozoospermia (6 to 12 million motile sperm/ml) (Yovich & Stanger, 1984).

Hereditary and genetic problems

Gene identification and sex selection of embryos in sex-linked disorders are just becoming possible with a huge potential to produce healthy babies in the future.

Acceptance

Many couples are childless by choice and have a satisfactory and happy relationship. Many childless couples, without the distraction of their own, have given a great deal of their time, energy and wisdom to other people's children with lasting benefit and consequent self-fulfilment. Nieces, nephews, god-children, neighbours' children can all fill the role. Children are a life-long commitment and responsibility but they can be a drain on personal and financial reserves. Remaining childless offers freedom and independence and a chance to develop skills, interests and careers which might be difficult to pursue when children have to take priority. This concept is probably more acceptable to couples who are older or have undergone some years of infertility treatment without success. Nevertheless, acceptance has a place in initial counselling.

Fostering

The temporary nature of fostering makes it less attractive to infertile couples. Children usually leave to return to their homes or go to an adoptive home. However, where a child has been fostered for 5 years or more, foster parents have the right to apply to the courts for an adoption hearing although there is no guarantee that adoption will be permitted. Many couples find fostering a most rewarding experience (Chennells & Hammond, 1990).

Adoption

Adoption is perceived by many couples as a poor option. Few babies are available and a baby is what they want. Many believe that, by the time their names come to the top of the waiting list for consideration, they will be unacceptably old. Some express distaste at the intrusion into their lives of the vetting procedure and the hurt they would feel if they were rejected. A number of authorities will not accept couples onto their waiting list while they are undergoing infertility investigations and treatment, which many couples consider unfair. Some of these fears are justified. In a recent report submitted to the Sheffield Family and Community Services Committee (Young, 1989) it is made clear to prospective adopters that, if they want to adopt a young baby from a straightforward background, it is unlikely that their application will be successful. In Sheffield, a city of 560 000 population, from April 1988 to March 1989, 12 healthy white babies under 6 months and 3 healthy black babies under 6 months were accepted for adoption.

Adoption agencies need applicants to be flexible both about the age of the child and the complexity of its background as many of the older children may have suffered physical or sexual abuse. There is an urgent need for adopters who are able to take children over the age of 5 years or to take family groups, but this is often a daunting prospect for couples who do not already have children of their own. Adoption policy is to place black or mixed race babies with similar parents so black or mixed race couples are particularly welcome to adoption agencies.

In the United Kingdom, the British Agencies for Adoption and Fostering (BAAF) are able to give detailed information about adoption and fostering throughout the country (Chennells & Hammond, 1990).

Adoption from abroad is a possibility but is both time consuming and expensive. A couple who adopted a baby from Brazil confirm it is not an option for the faint-hearted. The babies have usually been abandoned or badly neglected and may be in urgent need of medical attention. The paperwork can take many months with references and social workers' reports having to be translated into the language of the country concerned. It costs a great deal of money not only in legal and medical fees but also for the flights and accommodation. Only a few days' notice is given to come and collect the baby but it is not possible to leave the country until adoption procedures have been completed. That experience in Brazil took 5 weeks. However, for this particular couple, it was so successful that 12 months later they went back for another baby!

An organization called 'STORK' (STORK, 9 Woodland Green, Upton St Leonards, Gloucester GL4 8BD) is a national association of parents who have adopted children from other countries. It is not an adoption agency (no agency as yet deals with intercountry adoption in the UK), but members are willing to share their experiences with prospective adoptive parents who are still undecided about taking this step.

Donor insemination

Donor insemination (DI) is considered the appropriate form of treatment in a variety of conditions. Most commonly, the man is azoospermic or severely oligozoospermic; sperm motility may be very poor (asthenozoospermia) or there may be a large percentage of abnormal sperm forms present (teratozoospermia). The presence of a large number of antibody coated sperm may be another indication. Sterility may be the result of medical treatment (leukaemia, Hodgkin's disease) or surgical intervention (malignant testes, vasectomy, failed vasectomy reversal). Couples with normal fertility may seek donor insemination on account of hereditary disease (Huntington's chorea, polycystic kidneys) or following fatal genetic abnormalities in an earlier pregnancy (Werdnig–Hoffman disease). In the author's clinic, 36% of couples are considered suitable for DI on the basis of the male partner's semen profile. Knowledge of the variety of conditions where DI may be indicated can help couples put their own problem in perspective.

One of the attractions of DI is that the couple goes through a pregnancy and labour together as in normal conception and the baby carries the wife's genes. However, the decision to use semen from an unidentified donor to produce a much wanted child is not one to be taken lightly. The donation of gametes cannot be compared to the donation of blood and most people would agree that in-depth counselling is essential before this form of treatment is begun. The Human Fertilisation and Embryology Act, 1990 (HFE Act), makes it a condition that the couple be given 'a suitable opportunity to receive proper counselling about the implications of the proposed steps and have been provided with such relevant information as is proper'. At the moment, counselling for assisted reproduction is often done on a rather *ad hoc* basis with variable quality and content, but this should change with the Human Fertilization and Embryology Authority (HFE Authority) being under obligation to monitor the quality of counselling services. The licensing authority assumed its role with publication of its Code of Practice on 1 August 1991. It requires careful reading to ensure implementation of all its recommendations.

The British Infertility Counselling Association (BICA) was set up in 1988 by a group of professionals involved in different capacities with infertile people and aware of their needs. It hopes to be able to make recommendations for training, and to play an important role in the future development of infertility services.

Counselling for donor insemination

Couple referral

A good DI counsellor becomes a more effective one when the clinical services to which the couple are exposed are of a high standard with well-informed clinicians and sensitive clinic and nursing staff. Couples need a detailed explanation of their problem, from the referring doctor, which they can understand, and a chance to put their problem into perspective before they are referred. This is particularly so where the counsellors involved are not medically qualified. Laboratory services are equally important and must provide accurate, reliable tests of semen parameters. Clinicians involved in infertility programmes should be able to interpret the results and know the limitations of semen laboratory data to give a realistic fertility prognosis, thus avoiding inappropriate referral.

Counsellors should feel that the DI service under discussion offers the best possible chance of a conception. This implies a large pool of vigorously screened and well-counselled donors, high post-thaw motility and sperm samples with good fertilizing capacity. With that confidence, the counsellor can concentrate on the needs of the couple, the treatment and its implications.

Most DI clinics would prefer to treat married couples, or couples cohabiting over several years where the parents have a loving commitment to each other so that any child conceived grows up within a stable family unit. However, McCartney (1985) conducting psychiatric interviews on 12 single women seeking DI compared her findings with that of Merritt &

Steiner (1984) studying 100 single mothers conceiving naturally or adopting and concluded that comfortable effective parenting is possible for these women, although Frank & Brackley (1989) describe 'feelings of aloneness and vulnerability' in these women. The HFE Act (1990) states that 'A woman shall not be provided with treatment services unless account has been taken of the welfare of any child who may be born as a result of the treatment (including the needs of that child for a father)'. This may make it very difficult for single women, keen to become mothers using donor semen, to be treated at DI clinics.

Couple needs

Counsellors should be aware that the needs of the individuals may be different to their needs as a couple. (Husband/male partner are synonymous in this text.)

Men

Men need to come to terms with their infertility, be confident of their sense of male identity and have reached acceptance that, although not carrying their DNA, the child will be theirs in every other respect. Feelings of isolation can be helped when couples realize the number of people world-wide who are prepared to consider donor insemination as an option for them. The Royal College of Obstetricians and Gynaecologists which collates figures from DI clinics in the UK stated that 3562 couples were referred for treatment, and 1533 babies were born as a result of treatment in 1988. Every year 30 000 DI babies are born in the USA (OTA, 1987). In France, within the Federation CECOS, there were 3525 pregnancies during 1988–89 (Le Lannou & Lansac, Chapter 11). Enquiries regarding frequency of sexual intercourse or difficulties with erection or ejaculation may suggest the need for psychosexual counselling, and the couple should be referred as necessary. From experience, this is usually dealt with before DI is considered.

The fear of being unable to accept a DI child as truly his own is a worry that is often expressed by the male partner and this may delay the couple's decision-making and, on occasion, prevent them from proceeding. Where there are anxieties or doubts, it is often helpful to encourage them to talk to someone else: a member of their family or close friend who would respect their confidence or, if that is unacceptable, another couple who has already achieved a pregnancy with DI and is happy to share their experiences, may provide the necessary reassurance. It should then be left to the couple themselves to contact the counsellor if, and when, they feel ready to pursue discussions so there is no pressure to come to a decision.

Women

Women have to face the problem that the child they so desire is not going to have the genetic input of a much loved partner. They want their husband's baby, and using sperm from an unknown donor in order to become a mother can cause much heart-searching. It helps to point out that the personal input of a father and the loving environment in which a child grows up can make as significant a contribution to the child as the genes it carries. Some women are so desperate for a child that the husband is carried along as a reluctant participant. One must be alerted to this possibility where the woman does all the talking and her husband is monosyllabic or avoids eye contact. Opportunity should be provided to talk to the man on his own to allow him to express his feelings.

Women are naturally concerned about carrying a baby conceived with sperm from an unknown donor. A small proportion voice worries that sperm from a donor of a different race may be used inadvertently with distressing consequences; the risk of contracting AIDS is a common anxiety. It is reassuringly helpful to describe exactly how donors are recruited, rejected or accepted, the screening undertaken, the labelling and dating of straws, 6 months' quarantine for all semen samples with regular HIV checks on all donors and double checking the identity of all straws at the time of treatment.

The couple

The status of the DI child has long been a source of anxiety. In the UK before 1987, the child was considered to be illegitimate and expected to be registered with 'father unknown' on the birth certificate and sub-sequently adopted by the couple. In practice, this unrealistic action was rarely carried out, and probably virtually all the men registered them-selves as the father. However, in 1987, the Family Law Reform Act was introduced into Parliament, Section 27 of which provides that a child which is conceived as a result of DI should be recognized in law as being the husband's child provided the husband consented to the insemination. This situation also applies in about half the states in the USA and in some other jurisdictions, e.g. Canada and Australia (Cusine, 1989). Surprisingly, this did not include Scotland until the HFE Act (1990) became law. According to the HFEA Code of Practice where a woman is being treated together with a male partner and is unmarried or judicially separated, the male partner is considered the legal father of any resulting child and where possible consent to treatment should be obtained from the couple.

It is important that the couple recognize that their fertility problem may not be one-sided. A considerable number will have additional female problems diagnosed or undiagnosed, and this very much affects the prognosis for pregnancy (Chauhan *et al.*, 1989*a*). Donor insemination should be seen as a treatment for the couple. Husbands should never be excluded but encouraged to feel involved. Where possible they should accompany their wives when they attend and be present during the treatment if they so wish. Some clinics will allow husbands to perform the insemination under supervision and, where it has been offered, this has been taken up with enthusiasm. Some clinics have the facilities which allow husbands to treat their wives at home with encouraging results (McLaughlin *et al.*, 1983). Although the British Pregnancy Advisory Service (BPAS) has recently announced their withdrawal from DI, 30% of their DI was done at home: this may make the procedure much less stressful. Anxiety would appear to affect conception rates (Demyttenaere *et al.*, 1988) and, from experience, where couples seek DI because of genetic problems, previously highly fertile women can often take many months to conceive, and need an enormous amount of support and reassurance. The stress that the DI procedure may occasion the female has been largely neglected (Edelmann, 1989).

Confidentiality and secrecy

These are words that have always been associated with DI. As opposed to adoption, secrecy is easy to achieve because the woman becomes pregnant and the assumption is that it is her husband's. In the past, the attitude has been that, the less other people know, the better and easier for all concerned, including the child. Increasingly, as male infertility and DI become subjects frequently discussed by the media, the need for secrecy does not seem so obvious and more couples are willing to discuss DI with their family and friends, and to seek their support. However, many are convinced their families couldn't cope and would be hurtful and critical. Sadly, this is true, and divulging such information can be counterproductive. One couple had so many abusive phone calls from the husband's large family that they asked for an ex-directory line! Fortunately most families are extremely supportive and encouraging. Around 50% of couples will probably have discussed their intention to consider DI with at least one other non-medical person by the time they come for their first counselling appointment, but no more than 25% will have considered the possibility of telling the child in the future. About 10% will state, at first contact, that they intend telling the child, and are keen for guidance about the best time to start such discussions. There are two situations where most counsellors would agree children *must* be told: first where many members of the family and friends already know and the child might find out from someone other than his parents; secondly, where DI is preferred because of hereditary disease in the husband's family, or because a previous child has died of a genetic disease which carries a high risk of recurrence. In the future, reassurance will be needed that these problems have not been passed on. Otherwise, couples should be allowed to decide what is in the best interests of their child within their own particular family situation, but only where adequate counselling allows the couple to seriously consider the options of 'telling' or 'not telling'.

Telling the child

If couples are to be encouraged to tell their children of their conception by DI they are going to need guidance about when, how and what to tell the child. The best time from experience of workers with adoption is probably around 4–5 years or when the child first starts asking questions about how babies are made. Snowdens' book *Gift of a Child* (1984*b*) makes helpful suggestions and provides reassuring examples of the positive reaction of children told while in their late teens or early 20s but it would be wrong to assume that all children would accept such information with equanimity particularly in that age-group. *How I began* (NSW Infertility Social Workers Group, 1988) an Australian publication, seems to be written more for the 8–10 year age-group and includes a sex education aspect which is informative, but perhaps too explicit for a younger child. A small book entitled *My Story* attractively illustrated and written in a simple way for a 4–5 year old by two mothers of DI children is also available (Infertility Research Trust, Sheffield, 1991).

Couples should also have the assurance that help and support will be available when they are ready to talk to their children. Ideally, they should be able to come back to the clinic where they were treated for an exchange of information and ideas not only with familiar clinic staff but also with other couples in a similar situation.

It needs to be stressed that a child cannot be told something as important as this in isolation. Family and friends must also know so that when the child mentions it, which is bound to happen sooner or later, the response is happy and enthusiastic; this includes the teacher at playgroup or primary school as they are often the recipient of the confidences of their young pupils!

Where couples say they intend telling the children but have not yet mentioned it to their families or friends, it can be helpful to suggest that it is probably more appropriate to tell them once a pregnancy is confirmed and well established. After all, not every woman participating in DI treatment gets pregnant, and constant enquiries from sympathetic yet concerned family can be stressful. Once the baby arrives, many couples have found it too difficult to break the news and it only gets harder as the months and years go by.

Not telling the child

Some couples are adamant that 'not telling' is in the child's best interest. Like most parents they have a natural desire to protect their child from potential problems that might arise. They cite the possible frustration and anger at being unable to trace their natural father or their true paternal roots, the unkind, cruel taunts of other children and the anxiety that they might consider themselves oddities. Where there are several grandchildren in the family, couples often worry that their children might not receive as much love and attention as the others. Most men would also admit to the understandable fear that, if the child were told that 'Daddy' was not its real father, it might not love him as much. These are legitimate points but they must be weighed against the fact that many children would prefer their parents to be honest with them. Explained in a loving, caring way, and realizing what their parents went through to bring them into the world, it is more likely to bring the family closer together than cause alienation. In a society where one in three marriages end in divorce, many children are not brought up by their natural fathers, so comparisons with other children are less relevant. There is also the undisputed fact that secrets make one vulnerable and secrets from those one loves can be particularly hard to keep.

Whatever they decide to do, couples in the UK need to be aware of the changes in the law expressed in the HFE Act, Cl 31, which states that the licensing authority is to keep a register of:

1. all persons to whom infertility services including DI have been provided;
2. persons whose gametes are stored or used;
3. persons born as a consequence of such treatments.

At the age of 18 years, or 16 if planning to marry, persons can apply to the licensing authority for information if they think they may have been conceived by means of donor gametes. If the claim is justified, and after careful counselling of the implications of such a request, information may be given, but the identity of the donor will remain confidential. If the regulations governing the identity of the donor were to change in the future, it is clearly stated that these will not be made retrospective. However, in the event of any child being born with a congenital disability where civil liability proceedings were considered justifiable, the identity of the donor could be ordered by the court. Where there is the chance of consanguinity through marriage, information regarding donor gamete conceptions, where relevant, may be released, although what advice is to be offered where a couple have a common father is not indicated. It has been calculated that, if 2000 children are born by DI each year in the UK, and if each donor fathers five children, the possibility of a consanguineous marriage is unlikely to occur more than once in 50–100 years (Glass, 1960). There is no doubt that many children are not the offspring of their assumed fathers (McLaren & Parkes, 1973; Curie-Cohen, 1980), so inbreeding must occur unwittingly in the general population, increasing the risk of recessive disease. To ensure that DI does not add to this risk, it has been calculated that pregnancies per donor should not exceed 292 (Curie-Cohen, 1980); a number far greater than has ever been reported or imagined. Although there is a natural inclination to advocate restriction, these figures do not provide scientific justification for this practice. Increasing requests for DI and the ability to freeze sperm has made treatment more accessible and encouraged expansion of the service. Surplus semen straws are often distributed to different parts of the country, indeed the world, particularly to areas where donor recruitment may be more of a problem, so it may become important not to restrict the number of pregnancies unnecessarily. The HFEA has restricted the number of pregnancies to 10 but allowance has been made for more than one child of any donor being born into the same family, an increasingly possible and popular option.

Treatment

Couples are naturally keen to know how the insemination is performed, how a particular donor is chosen for them, and what chance they have of achieving a pregnancy. This should be discussed during the initial counselling session.

Clinics vary in the investigations required of the female before DI treatment is offered, from none at all, provided the woman has a regular menstrual cycle, to a more comprehensive assessment. This may include a biphasic temperature chart, cervical mucus awareness, a 21 day plasma progesterone level >18 nmol/l, a normal hysterosalpingogram (HSG) and/or a normal laparoscopy. Where the minimum of investigations is performed initially, most clinics would recommend an HSG or laparoscopy if the woman failed to conceive after 6 months. A history which suggests endometriosis or previous pelvic inflammatory disease would indicate the need for an early laparoscopy. Irregular, anovulatory cycles should be diagnosed and treated by the referring doctor before the couple reaches the counsellor.

Details of treatment, follow-up, pregnancy rates and a realistic treatment time should be discussed during the counselling sessions. Couples should be reminded that a pregnancy cannot be guaranteed. Most clinics would quote an overall 50% pregnancy rate. Where the man is azoospermic and his partner considered of normal fertility, the rate is closer to 80%. A treatment period of 9 months should be considered reasonable as many fertile couples can take that time to conceive.

Understandably, most couples would prefer a donor who matched the husband's physical characteristics as closely as possible. Matching is confined to height, build, hair and eye colour. Blood groups are matched where possible or particularly requested or when the woman is Rhesus negative. Many clinics will only use a cytomegalovirus (CMV) negative donor for a CMV negative woman to avoid passing on this infection to the fetus.

It cannot be emphasized too strongly that women undergoing DI should be treated as individuals. If a woman says she knows when she ovulates, she probably does, and treatment times can be calculated accordingly. Many women complain of receptionists giving appointments over the telephone based on nothing more than the days they were treated the previous month. These women are very sensitive, and the information they are given should match their level of understanding. A flexible approach is much more likely to be effective than a rigid, uncompromising 'we know best' attitude. At all times, they should feel able to share their anxieties about their treatment regimes with the nursing and medical staff involved.

Timing of inseminations is carried out effectively for the majority of women by recording basal body temperature and looking for ovulatory mucus. It may be worth mentioning that, if timing becomes difficult LH urinary dip-sticks, LH blood levels and follicular scanning can be used.

All treatment cycles should be reviewed by an experienced member of the medical staff, and appropriate suggestions and changes made as required. Good liaison between the nurses performing the inseminations and the doctors in charge of the clinic is essential, giving the women undergoing treatment the confidence they need. No couple should undergo months of treatment unsuccessfully without an opportunity to discuss with the doctor the possible reasons for failure and the options for the future. Options, including acceptance, adoption, or fostering, may then be easier to consider and other forms of treatment should also be discussed including *in vitro* fertilization (IVF), gamete intra-fallopian transfer (GIFT) and ovulatory stimulation and the appropriate referrals made.

The donors

Donor anonymity

The anonymity of donors is a controversial question. In 1985, the Swedish Government passed a law stating that the identity of the semen donor should be recorded to enable the child at the age of 18 years to contact the biological father. This resulted in the almost total disappearance of DI in Sweden and frequent referral of couples to other parts of Scandinavia (Hamberger, 1986) Three years later Bygdeman (1989) summed up the effect of the law. There had been a considerable decrease in the number of couples treated. Many hospitals no longer offered the service, mainly because the recruitment of donors became more difficult. Others like the Department of Obstetrics and Gynaecology at the Karolinska Hospital in Stockholm continued to provide a normal service, as the publicity which the insemination law received in the media allowed a sufficient number of donors to be recruited. However, this clinic only treats 20–25 women per year and can only offer four treatment cycles to each women. The number of donors in use at any one time varies between six and eight and six pregnancies are allowed per donor (Professor M. Bygdeman, personal communication). The number of couples choosing DI in Sweden declined presumably because they did not wish the child to be able to identify the donor, but also because many of them sought treatment in other countries.

In New Zealand, from a survey of 37 semen donors, Daniels (1987) stated that anonymity as a donor was *VERY* important for 68% and important for a further 27%. Donors were asked if they would still donate if children could trace their identity: 46% said they would not, 24% said they would and 30% were unsure. It must be stated that this is the reaction to a hypothetical situation and the reaction to a *de facto* situation might be different. A more recent UK survey (Robinson *et al.*, 1990) questioned 52 donors; 50% would be willing to have their identity released but it was noted that new donors appeared more anxious to maintain confidentiality than established donors. This suggests that, like the Swedish experience, if the identification of donors became law, recruitment would become a major problem.

Counselling of donors

Once donors have been carefully screened and selected, it is important that they have the chance to discuss the implications and responsibilities of becoming a semen donor with the opportunity to ask questions. Donors play the most important role in any DI clinic. The service cannot be offered without them, and they need to know they are part of a caring, responsible team who work to high standards of integrity and that no less is expected of them.

It is always illuminating for donors to realize the incidence of male infertility. At least one in six couples has difficulty in conceiving, and 24% of them will have significant male problems (Hull *et al.*, 1985). Equally interesting for them is to know the variety of problems where DI is offered as a treatment.

A personal and close family medical history should be discussed with particular reference to the more common congenital abnormalities (spina bifida, fibrocystic disease, Down's syndrome).

Despite vigorous screening, including karyotyping, spontaneous abortions and congenital abnormalities still occur in DI pregnancies but no more frequently than is found in normal conceptions (Lansac & Grefen-stette, 1990).

Screening of donors

The possibility of passing on a sexually transmitted disease (STD) during donor insemination should be given serious consideration, and homosex-uals and men using intravenous drugs, where there is an increased risk of developing AIDS (HIV infection), should always be rejected. Donors should be advised that any symptoms suggestive of infection which occur while they are participating in a donor programme must be reported and investigated in the best interests of the recipients as well as in their own and their partner's. As a reminder, donors should be required to sign a form confirming that they are free of infection including genital warts and herpes, with every donation. Once donations are complete, donors should attend the genito-urinary medicine clinic again for re-screening and all samples discarded if infection is present (see Chapter 2). Six months after the last donation, donors should be re-tested for HIV antibodies and, if negative, only then should the semen samples be released for patient use.

The American Fertility Society (1990) remains ambivalent about the use of CMV positive donors in an insemination programme. If they were to be excluded, this would cause an unacceptable drop in the number of suitable donors. Chauhan *et al.* (1989*b*) found that, in one particular clinic, 40% of the donors were CMV positive. At the same time, 30% of the recipient couples were both CMV positive, 35% were both negative, and in 35% only one member of the partnership was CMV positive. No one knows the frequency of latent CMV excretion in the semen of CMV positive men with the consequent risk of transmitting the infection to a recipient (see Chapter 2). Skinner and Billstrom (personal communi-cation) looked at four post-thaw ejaculate samples produced at different times over several months by ten CMV positive donors, and were unable to find CMV in any of the cultures. Until the extent of the risk is better known, it would seem reasonable to restrict the use of CMV positive donors to the treatment of women who are also CMV positive.

Reassurance should also be given to the donors that couples seeking DI are themselves carefully screened and counselled to ensure, as far as possible, that the children will grow up in a happy and loving environ-ment.

Long-term effects of DI

The incidence of marital break-up in couples who have had children by DI is difficult to assess. With one in three marriages in Britain ending in divorce, there is no evidence that couples who have children with DI are more likely to separate than those within the normal population. Most clinics offering DI would offer the impression that divorce following DI is relatively rare (Snowden & Snowden, 1984*a*). Goebel and Lubke (1987) following up 96 couples 17 years after their DI treatment, found that, where the DI had been successful or where having failed, adoption had been successful, 10% of the couples were divorced. Where neither DI nor adoption had been successful, 35% were divorced. Bendvold *et al.* (1989) compared separation rates of women in Norway conceiving after DI with those conceiving normally, and concluded that the separation rate in DI families does not differ significantly from that of a demographically matched population.

A recent study in Australia (Kovacs *et al.*, 1990) assessed psychosocial behaviour in 22 DI children compared with 20 children conceived naturally and ten adopted children, matched by sex and age, and found no differences. An interesting observation emerged. The parents of each child completed the questionnaire with the social worker present. For the DI couples, the interview was with both parents, almost always, both actively participating; similarly with the adopted children. In contrast, almost all the interviews, where the children had been conceived naturally, were with the mother alone, as this was considered the mother's role. This might suggest that the fathers of children conceived by DI, contrary to what might be imagined, have much more commitment and involvement with their children than many natural fathers appear to have.

There is very little information available on the outcome of DI from either the parents' or the children's viewpoint. This is due mainly to the secrecy which has tended to enshroud the procedure in the past, and more documentation is required to encourage awareness and understanding.

DI, the future

If the donor insemination services on offer to infertile couples are to be improved, much more consideration must be given to their needs and expectations, to the involvement of the donors and to the long-term future of the children conceived.

Semen donors need to be given more prominence. A greater awareness of their role in the DI process will help engender a responsible and reliable attitude to what they are doing, and they should also be given the opportunity to express their feelings and encouraged to ask questions.

Counselling which provides information, support and the opportunity to discuss long-term implications is seen as essential not only by the couples themselves and the professionals working in the field but also by society in the form of the Government's Human Fertilization and Embryology Act.

A baby should not be seen as the end-point but as the beginning of a long-term relationship, and couples need reminding that babies grow up, developing through childhood and adolescence into adulthood. More couples seem willing to discuss their male fertility problems openly and honestly, but many still feel, quite sincerely, that secrecy is in the best interests of the child. The general population is neither well informed nor sympathetic, so 'open' policies must be linked with education from an early age about the realities of infertility. This is an area which merits much more thought and discussion.

DI is not a treatment for male infertility, but a substitution, and the aim for DI clinics in the future should be to consider not only refinement of the service they offer but development of ideas which will eventually allow effective treatment to replace DI for the vast majority of couples.

References

American Fertility Society. (1990). New guidelines for the use of semen donor insemination. *Fertility and Sterility*, **53** Suppl 1.

Bendvold, E., Skjaeraasen, J., Moe, N., Sjoberg, D. & Kravdal, O. (1989). Marital break-up among couples raising families by artificial insemination by donor. *Fertility and Sterility*, **51**, 980–3.

Berger, D. M. (1980). Reactions to male infertility and donor insemination. *American Journal of Psychiatry*, **137**, 1047–9.

Berger, D. M., Eisen, A., Shuber, J. & Doody, K. F. (1986). Psychological patterns in donor insemination couples. *Canadian Journal of Psychiatry*, **31**, 818–23.

BICA. (1988) c/o Social Work Department, St Bartholomew's Hospital, West Smithfield, London EC1A 7BE.

Bygdeman, M. (1989). Swedish law concerning insemination. *International Planned Parenthood Federation Medical Bulletin*, **23**, 3–4.

Chauhan, M., Barratt, C. L. R., Cooke, S. M. S. & Cooke, I. D. (1989a). Differences in the fertility of donor insemination recipients – a study to provide prognostic guidelines as to its success and outcome. *Fertility and Sterility*, **51**, 815–19.

Chauhan, M., Barratt, C. L. R., Cooke, S. & Cooke, I. D. (1989*b*). Screening for cytomegalovirus antibody in a donor insemination program: difficulties in implementing the American Fertility Society guidelines. *Fertility and Sterility*, **51**, 901–2.

Chennells, P. & Hammond, C. (1990). *Adopting a Child*, 3rd edn. London: British agencies for Adoption & Fostering.

Connolly, K. J., Edelmann, R. J. & Cooke, I. D. (1987). Distress and marital problems associated with infertility. *Journal of Reproductive and Infant Psychology*, **5**, 1–9.

Curie-Cohen, M. (1980). The frequency of consanguineous matings due to multiple use of donors in artificial insemination. *American Journal of Human Genetics*, **32**, 589–600.

Cusine, D. (1989). Legal issues in human reproduction. In *Legal Issues in Human Reproduction*, ed. S. McLean, pp. 17–44. Aldershot, England: Gower.

Daniels, K. R. (1987). Semen donors in New Zealand: their characteristics and attitudes. *Clinical Reproduction and Fertility*, **5**, 177–90.

Demyttenaere, K., Nijs, P., Steeno, O., Koninckx, P. & Evers-Kiebooms, G. (1988). Anxiety and conception rates in donor insemination. *Journal of Psychosomatic Obstetrics and Gynaecology*, **8**, 175–81.

Edelmann, R. J. (1989). Psychological aspects of artificial insemination by donor. *Journal of Psychosomatic Obstetrics and Gynaecology*, **10**, 3–13.

Frank, D. I. & Brackley, M. H. (1989). The health experience of single women who have children through artificial donor insemination. *Clinical Nurse Specialist* (United States), **3**, 156–60.

Glass, D. V. (1960). Quoted in *Report of the Departmental Committee on Human Artificial Insemination*. London, HMSO.

Goebel, P. & Lubke, F. (1987). Catamnestic study of 96 couples with heterologous insemination. *Geburtshilfe und Frauenheilkunde*, **47**, 636–40.

Hamberger, L. (1986). Artificial insemination by donor (AID) in Sweden. *Human Reproduction*, **1**, 49.

Hendry, W. F. (1988). Role of urological surgery. In *Advances in Clinical Andrology*, C. L. R. Barratt and I. D. Cooke, eds, pp. 31–47, Lancaster, England: MTP Press Ltd.

Hendry, W. F., Hughes, L., Scammell, G., Pryor, J. P. & Hargreave, T. B. (1990). Comparison of prednisolone and placebo in subfertile men with antibodies to spermatozoa. *Lancet*, **i**, 85–8.

Hull, M. G. R., Glazener, C. M. A., Kelly, N. J., Conway, D. I., Foster, P. A., Hinton, R. A., Coulson, C., Lambert, P. A., Watt, E. M. & Desai, K. M. (1985). Population study of causes, treatment, and outcome of infertility. *British Medical Journal*, **291**, 1693–7.

Human Fertilisation and Embryology Act. (1990). London: HMSO.

Humphrey, M. & Humphrey, H. (1987). Marital relationships in couples seeking donor insemination. *Journal of Biosocial Science*, **19**, 209–19.

Infertility Research Trust. (1991). *My Story*. J. W. Northend Ltd, Sheffield, 20 pp.

Jequier, A. M., Cummins, J. M., Gearon, C., Apted, S. L., Yovich, J. M. & Yovich, J. L. (1990). A pregnancy achieved using sperm from the epididymal caput in idiopathic obstructive azoospermia. *Fertility and Sterility*, **53**, 1104–5.

Kovacs, G. T., Mushin, D., Kane, H. & Baker, H. W. G. (1990). A controlled study of the psychosocial development of children conceived following insemination with donor semen. *Fertility Society of Australia Meeting*, Perth, Australia.

Lansac, J. & Grefenstette, I. (1990). La Grossesse apres l'IAD: evolution du conceptus. In *L'insemination artificielle*, CECOS, pp. 189–95. Paris: Masson.

McCartney, C. F. (1985). Decision by single women to conceive by artificial donor insemination. *Journal of Psychosomatic Obstetrics and Gynaecology*, **4**, 321–8.

McLaren, A. & Parkes, A. S. (1973). Legal and other aspects of artificial insemination by donor (AID) and embryo transfer. *Journal of Biosocial Science*, **5**, 205–8.

McLaughlin, E. A., Bromwich, P. D., Macken, A. M., Walker, A. P. & Newton, J. R. (1983). Use of home insemination in programmes of artificial insemination with donor semen. *British Medical Journal*, **287**, 1110.

Merritt, S. & Steiner, L. (1984). *And Baby Makes Two: Motherhood without Marriage*, pp. 264. New York: Franklin-Watts.

New South Wales Infertility Social Workers Group. (1988). *How I Began. The Story of Donor Insemination*, J. Paul, ed., Fertility Society of Australia.

Office of Technology and Assessment (OTA), Congress of the United States (1987). *Artificial Insemination: Practice in the United States*. US Government, Washington 1988 pp. 112.

Robinson, J. N., Forman, R. G., Clark, A., Egan, D., Dalton, J., Franklin, P. & Barlow, D. H. (1990). Anonymity of gamete donors: a survey of attitudes. *Journal of Reproduction and Fertility*, Abstract Series **5**, 67.

Silber, J. S., Balmaceda, J., Borrero, C., Ord, T. & Asch, R. (1988). Pregnancy with sperm aspiration from the proximal head of the epididymis: a new treatment for congenital absence of the vas deferens. *Fertility and Sterility*, **50**, 525–8.

Snowden, R. & Snowden, E. (1984*a*). The married couple and AID. In *The Gift of a Child*, pp. 63–73. London: George Allen & Unwin.

Snowden, R. & Snowden, E. (1984*b*). AID children. In *The Gift of a Child*, pp. 99–114. London: George Allen & Unwin.

Young, M.T. (1989). Annual report of the work of the Adoption Agency from April 1988–March 1989. *City of Sheffield Family and Community Services Department*.

Yovich, J. L. & Stanger, J. D. (1984). The limitations of *in vitro* fertilisation from males with severe oligospermia and abnormal sperm morphology. *Journal of in Vitro Fertilisation and Embryo Transfer*, **1**, 172–9.

4

Sperm transport in the female tract

J. W. OVERSTREET and E. Z. DROBNIS

Introduction

The goal of therapeutic donor insemination (DI) is to introduce adequate numbers of functional sperm at a time and location which will maximize the probability of conception. In spite of substantial scientific and clinical effort, the fecundability of patients in DI programs usually falls far short of natural fecundability (Barratt, Chauhan & Cooke, 1990). Because most DI programmes utilize cryopreserved sperm for insemination, a primary cause of this diminished fertility is the cryodamage sustained by human sperm during processing and preservation. The current thinking is that the root cause of cryodamage to sperm (Watson, 1985; Hammerstedt, Graham & Nolan, 1990), as well as other types of cells (see Mazur, 1984) is the breakdown of membrane permeability barriers. During cryopreservation, even if intracellular ice formation is avoided, many forces stress the membrane, including increased solute concentration accompanying intracellular dehydration, mechanical shear, osmotic damage during warming, and lipid phase separation (see Chapter 6 for further details.) Large increases in membrane permeability will render sperm immotile, but among the surviving motile cells, sublethal increases in permeability could have profound and diverse effects on sperm function. A substantial research effort is currently directed at understanding and mitigating the factors which result in sublethal cryodamage, and it is likely that these studies will provide improved cryopreservation methods in the future. In the meantime, substantial improvements in DI success may still be achieved by modifications and innovations in patient management and DI technique.

Fertilization in mammals is a highly regulated process that is dependent on the transport of physiologically competent spermatozoa to the upper

33

oviduct near the time of ovulation (Overstreet, 1983). An understanding of the physiology of spermatozoa in the female reproductive tract is essential for rational design of DI procedures and evaluation of their efficacy. Unfortunately, very little is known of human sperm biology *in vivo*. In recent years, even animal experiments have been limited, with major research in gamete biology being focussed at the cell and molecular level of investigation (Overstreet, Katz & Cross, 1988). It is logical to assume that the subfertility of cryodamaged sperm cells may be due in part to abnormality or inefficiency of their transport through the female tract. Thus, the ability to improve the technology of DI will be enhanced by a better understanding of sperm interaction with the female tract. In this chapter, current knowledge of sperm transport and sperm physiology in the female tract of humans and other mammals will briefly be reviewed. The limited clinical information which is available on the sequence of biological events which may follow DI will be discussed, together with how the natural processes may be perturbed by artificial insemination.

Sperm transport in the female reproductive tract

Insemination and passive sperm transport

Spermatozoa appear to reach the upper reproductive tract and/or peritoneal cavity within minutes of coitus in all mammalian species including humans (Overstreet, 1983). Because spermatozoa have been recovered from the human oviduct within five minutes of intracervical insemination (Settlage, Motoshima & Tredway, 1973), this rapid sperm transport is also likely to follow DI. The mechanism of rapid sperm transport is not well understood, but it may involve reflex-mediated muscular contractions of the female reproductive tract. Such contractions have been recorded during human coitus (Fox, Wolff & Baker, 1970). The phenomenon of rapid sperm transport has been studied most extensively in rabbits. Rabbits, like humans, ejaculate into the vagina during coitus. As in humans, rapid sperm transport follows artificial insemination as well as coital insemination (Overstreet & Cooper, 1978). In this model species, both physical and chemical stimuli appear to initiate the process, which is mediated by the autonomic nervous system (Overstreet & Tom, 1982). Although rabbit sperm have been recovered from the upper oviductal ampulla and peritoneal cavity within one minute of mating, the oviductal sperm were immotile and visibly disrupted (Overstreet & Cooper, 1978). The phenomenon of rapid sperm transport appeared to be of brief duration, and there was little evidence of sperm in the upper oviduct by 90 minutes post-coitus. Therefore, at least in rabbits, rapid sperm transport probably plays no direct role in fertilization. Experimental studies have been carried out with other laboratory species and with farm animals, in which the success of fertilization was examined after oviducts were ligated or transected from the uterus at different intervals after mating (Hunter, 1987). The results of these experiments also suggest that the functional sperm population may not reach the mammalian oviduct for several hours after mating (Hunter, 1987).

The widespread occurrence and apparent similarity of rapid sperm transport phenomena among mammals suggest that there is an important, although still unrecognized, biological function for this process. One possible function is the delivery of molecules from the sperm or seminal plasma that could serve as local messengers or signals to the female tract (Overstreet, 1983). Following DI, abnormalities of rapid sperm transport could contribute to reductions in fecundability.

There are data in the rabbit model which suggest how insemination techniques may elicit inappropriate responses from the female tract and thereby perturb normal reproductive physiology. Intrauterine insemination (IUI) is widely used in DI (Dodson & Haney, 1991; Corson & Kemmann, 1991). One logic for this approach is that the fertility of a relatively small number of fragile (cryodamaged) sperm cells will be enhanced by placing them nearer to the site of fertilization. There is evidence which suggests that cryopreserved human sperm may have a reduced ability to penetrate cervical mucus (Fjallbrant & Ackerman, 1969; Ulstein, 1972; Zavos & Cohen, 1980). Therefore, circumvention of the cervical barrier could be advantageous, in itself. While there are some clinical data suggesting that IUI may lead to higher fecundability after DI (Byrd *et al.*, 1990), there are no experiments which demonstrate the physiological basis for the presumed effectiveness of IUI. To the contrary, we found a lower fertilization rate (76% vs 98%) and a lower percentage of 4-cell embryos (17% v. 42%) among the fertilized oocytes when non-frozen rabbit sperm were inseminated with IUI in comparison with vaginal insemination (Overstreet & Bedford, 1976). Subsequent unpublished experiments revealed similar numbers of oviductal sperm after IUI and vaginal insemination, suggesting that the differences in fertilization rates could not be explained by differences in sperm numbers. It appears that the lower fertilization rates after IUI in these experiments may have been due to differences in sperm fertility and ultimately to female reproductive dysfunction.

In other unpublished experiments, sperm were recovered from the oviduct after different numbers of sperm were inseminated by IUI. Fifteen animals were inseminated surgically with 1×10^6 sperm in one uterine horn and 50×10^6 in the contralateral horn. Normally, only a few hundred sperm can be recovered from the rabbit oviductal ampulla 12 hours after insemination (Overstreet, Cooper & Katz, 1978), and more that 75% are progressively motile (Cooper, Overstreet & Katz, 1979). In four of fifteen animals receiving IUI, thousands of immotile sperm were present in the tubal ampulla, and in every case, the abnormal transport occurred on the side where 50×10^6 sperm were inseminated. Such large numbers of dead sperm are often found in the rabbit oviduct as a consequence of rapid sperm transport (Overstreet & Cooper, 1978), but rapid transport is over within minutes of coitus and no evidence of these sperm remains by 12 hours after insemination (Overstreet *et al.*, 1978). The presence of such sperm twelve hours after IUI is certainly abnormal and may be related to abnormal contractions of the uterus and oviducts. Only two of fifteen animals had any evidence of fertilization when 50×10^6 sperm were inseminated, but two fertilized eggs were recovered from one ampulla together with two thousand dead sperm (unpublished observations). Whether or not the rabbit is an appropriate model for gamete transport in women, these observations emphasize the need to evaluate critically biological assumptions (such as the fate of sperm after IUI) which are based on intuition rather than experimental evidence.

Sperm survival and migration in the female

After rapid transport, sperm migration through the female tract continues until the time of ovulation. During this period, sperm accumulate in various regions of the tract. Depending on the species, these sites include the vagina, the uterus and the lower oviduct. When insemination precedes ovulation by several hours, these regions probably serve as sites of sperm storage or reservoirs (Overstreet, 1983). In women, for example, viable sperm may be recovered from cervical mucus for as long as five days following insemination (Gould, Overstreet & Hanson, 1984). The anatomy of the female reproductive tract, and hence the biology of sperm accumulation in mammals, varies widely among species. Most mammals have intravaginal insemination at coitus, and in many species, including humans, the cervix functions as an effective anatomical block to passage of seminal plasma and most of the spermatozoa (Overstreet, 1983).

In primates and ruminants, the cervix is filled with mucus. This fluid has been considered to be important for sperm accumulation in sheep, cattle and goats (Hawk, 1987; Hunter, 1987), as well as in monkeys (Jaszczak & Hafez, 1973) and in women (Overstreet *et al.*, 1988). Immediately following coitus, spermatozoa can be found throughout the cervical mucus in women (Sobrero & MacLeod, 1962). Sperm entry into the cervix from the vagina may also continue for several hours, but the acidic vaginal environment does not promote prolonged sperm survival in humans. Measurements of sperm motility in cervical mucus after DI with non-frozen sperm have revealed no significant changes in swimming speed between one and forty-eight hours following insemination (Hanson & Overstreet, 1981). With the development of methods to recover sperm from mucus, the apparent interval of functional sperm longevity after DI was extended to eighty hours, because sperm of this age were able to penetrate the human zona pellucida (Gould *et al.*, 1984). The swimming speeds of sperm recovered from mucus appeared to diminish by 120 hours after insemination, but the velocities remained comparable to those of sperm freshly washed from seminal plasma (Gould *et al.*, 1984). Comparable data on cryopreserved sperm are not available, but the information which is available suggests that their longevity is substantially less than that of non-frozen sperm (see below).

There has been considerable debate concerning the location within the cervix where sperm may be stored (Overstreet & Katz, 1990). There is experimental evidence in ruminants which suggests that the cervical mucosa, rather than the cervical mucus itself, is the biologically important site of sperm accumulation (Mattner, 1966, 1968). Although there is only a limited evidence in humans which demonstrates accumulation of sperm in epithelial crypts of the cervical mucosa (Insler *et al.*, 1980), damage to sperm membranes during cryopreservation could impair their ability to migrate to these areas and/or to form appropriate interactions with the cervical epithelium. As mentioned above, vigorously motile cryopreserved sperm have a reduced ability to penetrate cervical mucus. The cause of this apparent dysfunction is unknown, but observations of the interaction between cervical mucus and abnormal, non-frozen sperm may provide some insights. Comparisons of sperm morphology in semen and in cervical mucus have suggested that the mucus acts as a biological filter, restricting entry of morphological abnormal sperm (Hanson & Overstreet, 1981). Many abnormal sperm are probably excluded from penetrating the semen–mucus interface because of dyskinetic motility (Feneux, Serres & Jouannet, 1985), and those abnormal sperm which

Table 4.1. *Sperm survival in cervical mucus after artificial insemination with donor semen*

Sperm preparation	Non-frozen sperm	Cryopreserved sperm	Cryopreserved sperm
Number of cycles	37	37	19
Number of hours after DI	48 h	48 h	24 h
Percentage of cycles with sperm survival	57%	19%	42%

Note: Insemination with cervical cup (see Hanson *et al.*, 1982).
Timing of insemination by basal body temperature.
Sperm survival was considered positive if any sperm were seen.

gain entry are further impeded by mucus resistance (Katz *et al.*, 1990). This increased resistance is probably related to abnormalities of the sperm surface which interfere with the close association between the sperm and the glycoproteins of the mucus microstructure (Yudin, Hanson & Katz, 1989). Sperm surface abnormalities resulting from cryodamage could have similar deleterious effects.

There is good evidence that the number of motile sperm observed in cervical mucus after insemination correlates with sperm concentration in the ejaculate (Tredway, Buchanan & Drake, 1978) and there is a significant association between sperm survival for 48 hours in cervical mucus and conception after DI with non-frozen sperm (Hanson, Overstreet & Katz, 1982). Sperm survive for a shorter time in the cervix after DI with cryopreserved sperm (Table 4.1), and this decreased longevity *in vivo* may explain the apparent efficacy of multiple daily inseminations when cryopreserved sperm are inseminated (Mahadevan *et al.*, 1982). A shorter period of sperm survival after cryopreservation is also consistent with the higher fecundability which has been reported when DI is well timed in relation to ovulation (Smith, Rodriguez-Rigau & Steinberger, 1981). Fecundability after DI with cryopreserved sperm appears to increase as the number of motile sperm in the inseminate increases (Millet & Jondet, 1980; Brown, Boone & Shapiro, 1988). The requirement for large numbers of motile sperm in DI may be attributed to poor sperm survival *in vivo* or to other manifestations of sublethal cryodamage in some or all of the sperm cells (see below). In fact, the necessity for increased numbers of cryopreserved sperm, as opposed to more

Table 4.2. *Retrograde sperm migration and prolonged sperm survival in cervical mucus (CM) after intra-uterine insemination (IUI)*

DI method	Number of women	Number of cycles	% Cycles with CM sperm at 48 h
AI-cup[a]	26[b]	229	21%
IUI	26[b]	106	43%

[a] Insemination with cervical cup (see Hanson *et al.*, 1982).
[b] Paired data for women receiving IUI because of poor sperm recovery from cervical mucus 48 hours after AI-cup (Clisham *et al.*, 1989*a*).

effectively preserved sperm, cannot be determined with existing data. In studies of sperm numbers and fecundability, the number of motile sperm in the inseminate may be confounded by two important factors: 1) individual donor, because the sperm of some donors freeze better than the sperm of other donors, and 2) day-to-day variations in freezing treatments. As a consequence, inseminates with fewer motile sperm may be those from donors with poor freezability and/or those which were processed on days when freezability was relatively poor. The remaining motile sperm in these inseminates may have sustained greater cryoda-mage, and this damage may affect their functional capacity. These effects can be evaluated with appropriately designed experiments, but such studies have not yet been reported.

In view of the shorter longevity of cryopreserved sperm and the apparent benefit of timing DI with ovulation, the use of IUI in this setting would appear to be advantageous. Experiments in animal models have raised questions regarding the fate of sperm after IUI (see above). Although clinical studies have suggested the efficacy of this approach (Byrd *et al.*, 1990), the biological basis of its effectiveness is not clear. The procedure does not bypass the cervix in a functional sense because sperm are frequently found in the cervical mucus after IUI (Table 4.2). A similar retrograde passage of uterine sperm has been observed following IUI in sheep (Lightfoot & Restall, 1971). It is possible that IUI may be effective in some cases because it leads to more efficient entry of sperm into cervical mucus. Nevertheless, there is insufficient biological and clinical information to draw any firm conclusions regarding the advantages versus disadvantages of IUI therapy.

There is considerable variation between species in the biology of sperm entry into the uterus. In species with cervical mucus, sperm probably cross an interface between the mucus and uterine fluid to reach the uterine lumen. Three dimensional reconstructions of the bovine cervical mucosa have suggested that longitudinal mucosal folds, which are continuous with the endometrium, may provide privileged paths for sperm migration along the epithelial surfaces (Mullins & Saacke, 1989). In rabbits, the cervix contains little mucus and the organ may act like a valve to restrict sperm migration to the uterus. Because rabbit sperm may live for many hours in the vagina, there may be continuous passage of sperm from the vagina to the uterus via the cervix (Overstreet *et al.*, 1978). In rodent species, horses, pigs and dogs, whole semen enters the uterus, and sperm passage across the cervix is the result of female visceral contractions and/or ejaculation. The balance of evidence indicates that in most species the uterus serves as more of a conduit for motile sperm than a regulator of sperm migration. The uterus may serve as a source of temporary sperm supply for the oviduct, and the uterotubal junction appears to be specialized to regulate sperm entry into the oviduct (Overstreet, 1983). The isthmus of the oviduct serves as a site of sperm retention in most mammals, including rabbits, rodents, pigs and ruminants (Overstreet, 1983). Although ruminants accumulate sperm in the oviductal isthmus as well as in the cervix, there is controversy concerning the relative importance of the two regions as sites of sperm storage (Hunter, 1987). There is no conclusive information on sperm accumulation in the primate oviduct, but histological studies of the oviducts of mated cynomolgus macaques have suggested that an isthmic sperm reservoir may also be present in non-human primates (Overstreet & VandeVoort, 1990). The previous observations of sperm in the human oviduct have not been made in such a way as to distinguish a site of sperm accumulation, if it exists.

Sperm physiology in the female tract

The physiological changes in sperm cells that are required for sperm migration to the oviduct and for fertilization are collectively termed capacitation (Yanagimachi, 1981, 1988). The kinetics of capacitation have been described for a number of mammalian species *in vitro* (Yanagimachi 1981, 1988) and *in vivo* (Bedford, 1970, 1983). Many changes have been detected in sperm cells during capacitation *in vitro* but the relationship of these cellular events to sperm physiology *in vivo* is poorly understood (Yanagimachi, 1981, 1988; Bedford, 1983). There is evidence that sperm transport and capacitation *in vivo* are interrelated (Overstreet, 1983; Bedford, 1983). This linkage may be critical for controlling the migration to the oviduct of sperm cells that are competent to fertilize, as well as for regulating entry of the fertilizing sperm into the oviductal ampulla during the periovulatory period.

It is generally believed that the acrosome reaction of the fertilizing sperm must take place at or near the zona pellucida, and the natural stimulus for this event may involve molecules associated with the occyte or its investments (Meizel 1985; Yanagimachi, 1988). The occurrence of acrosome reactions at inappropriate times or locations may be incompatible with fertilization. For example, observations of hamster gamete interaction *in vitro* have revealed that acrosome reacted sperm cannot initiate penetration of the cumulus investment (Drobnis & Katz, 1990). In some species, acrosome reacted sperm are unable to bind to the zona pellucida (Yanagimachi, 1988). Acrosomal damage is a common sequel of cryopreservation (Hammerstedt *et al.*, 1990), and there is evidence that acrosome reactions may occur spontaneously after thawing in viable, cryopreserved human sperm (Critser *et al.*, 1987). This manifestation of sublethal cryodamage may be an important cause of diminished fertility after DI with cryopreserved sperm.

Prolonged acrosomal stability of sperm *in vivo* and a uniformity of their response to capacitation conditions may be required to ensure that sperm reaching the oocyte are competent to fertilize, regardless of their period of residence in the female tract. Human sperm that are recovered from cervical mucus into a non-capacitating medium can penetrate the human zona pellucida and fuse with zona-free hamster oocytes (Lambert *et al.*, 1985). Thus, it appears that human sperm capacitation can be initiated, if not completed, in the cervix. Because capacitation can be defined operationally as the physiological prerequisites of the acrosome reaction (Yanagimachi, 1988), the capacitation status of human sperm can be examined by challenge with biological agonists of the acrosome reaction. Both human follicular fluid (Suarez, Wolf & Meizel, 1986) and solubilized human zona pellucida (Cross *et al.*, 1988) have been used for this purpose. This approach was used in recent experiments with cervical mucus collected after DI with non-frozen sperm (Zinaman *et al.*, 1989). The mucus was incubated in BWW culture medium and the sperm were allowed to 'swim out' of the mucus and into the medium for subsequent incubation *in vitro*. The cervical sperm could be induced to acrosome react in response to follicular fluid after 6 hours of incubation. In more recent studies, acrosome reactions have been observed in response to follicular fluid as early as 2 1/2 hours after migration from mucus (Overstreet & Davis, 1992). This capacitation interval is very short in comparison with other systems for sperm capacitation *in vitro*, which may require 24 hours of incubation before sperm will acrosome react in response to follicular fluid (Suarez *et al.*, 1986; Zinaman *et al.*, 1989). The time requirement for acrosomal response to follicular fluid appears to be independent of sperm age in the reproductive tract, because similar results were obtained with sperm recovered between 1 hour and 72 hours after DI (Zinaman *et al.*, 1989). These findings support the concept that there is conservation of sperm function in the cervix, and they are consistent with the notion of a cervical sperm reservoir.

Ongoing studies of cryopreserved sperm have provided evidence of sperm dysfunction in the cervical environment which may lead to diminished fertility after DI. In these experiments, cryopreserved sperm were recovered from cervical mucus 24 hours after DI, and were tested for acrosomal status and capacitation kinetics by the same methods previously used for non-frozen sperm (Clisham *et al.*, 1989b; Drobnis *et al.*, 1990). In contrast to non-frozen sperm, cryopreserved sperm acrosome reacted in response to follicular fluid after only 1 hour incubation (12% *v* 2% for non-frozen sperm) and spontaneously acrosome reacted without exposure to agonist following 6 hours incubation (11% v. 3% for non-frozen sperm). These findings demonstrate a functional difference between cryopreserved sperm and non-frozen sperm that was manifested as a result of interaction with the female tract. This apparent increase in acrosomal lability may result in premature acrosome reactions in the female tract, which may be responsible, at least in part, for the decreased fertility of cryopreserved sperm.

Sperm capacitation in cervical mucus may be initiated by shearing of seminal plasma components from the sperm surface during physical interaction between the sperm and the mucus microstructure (Overstreet *et al.*, 1992). The primary importance of sperm–mucus interaction in this process is indicated by studies of sperm capacitation kinetics after exposure to cervical mucus *in vitro*. The same duration of incubation *in vitro* was required, and the same acrosomal response to follicular fluid was observed, whether sperm were recovered after DI or were allowed to migrate through cervical mucus in vitro (Zinaman *et al.*, 1989). In paired experiments, cryopreserved sperm were challenged with follicular fluid after penetration of cervical mucus *in vitro* or after recovery from the reproductive tract 24 hours following DI. In each experiment, the acrosomal physiology of sperm recovered from the cervix was predicted by the *in vitro* test (Drobnis *et al.*, 1990). These findings indicate that *in vitro* tests of sperm–cervical mucus interaction may be useful tools for developing improved cryopreservation methods.

Capacitated sperm *in vivo* and *in vitro* undergo changes in their movement characteristics from that of linear, forwardly progressive motion to that of less linear, vigorous, hyperactivated motility. Hyperactivation was first described in hamster sperm (Gwatkin & Anderson, 1969; Yanagimachi, 1969) and has subsequently been observed in other laboratory animal and domestic species as well as in humans (Katz *et al.*, 1989; Drobnis & Katz, 1991). Hyperactivation is considered to be an important marker of capacitation, and may be necessary to produce the forces required for sperm migration and fertilization in mammalian species (Katz *et al.*, 1989; Katz & Drobnis, 1990). Hyperactivation of human sperm motility has been reported under capacitation conditions using a variety of technical approaches including visual observations (Burkman, 1984), high speed videomicrography (Morales *et al.*, 1988), and computer aided sperm analysis (CASA) (Robertson, Wolf & Tash, 1988). CASA techniques have been used to demonstrate a temporal correlation between hyperactivation and the occurrence of the acrosome reaction in human sperm (Robertson *et al.*, 1988). Advanced CASA techniques involving multivariate statistical approaches and cluster analyses have revealed subpopulations of sperm with apparent hyperactivation following migration from cervical mucus (Overstreet & Davis, 1992). These techniques provide a potential means of detecting defects or changes in sperm physiology. In the future, they may be used together with acrosome reaction agonists to further investigate capacitation abnormalities and acrosomal dysfunction in cryopreserved sperm.

Little is known of sperm physiology in the human uterus or oviducts. The sperm capacitation phenomena in the uterus and oviducts have been studied extensively in model species (Bedford, 1970, 1983; Moore & Bedford, 1983). For example, the role of the female's endocrine status and the relative efficiency of capacitation in the uterus versus the oviducts have been determined. However, the relevance of these model systems to human sperm physiology is uncertain. As previously discussed, the lower isthmus of the oviduct appears to function as a sperm reservoir in many species. Accumulation of sperm in the oviductal isthmus is aided by mechanical factors such as the narrow lumen which may be filled with a mucus-like secretion (Jansen, 1980). The ciliary beat and muscular contractions of this region are directed primarily toward the uterus

(Overstreet, 1983). Sperm retention in the lower isthmus of the rabbit oviduct is associated with reversible cessation of flagellar activity (Burkman, Overstreet & Katz, 1984) and sperm adherence to epithelial surfaces (Cooper *et al.*, 1979). Similar phenomena may occur in the mouse (Suarez, 1987) and hamster (Smith, Koyanagi & Yanagimachi, 1988). The cellular mechanisms by which the female tract can immobilize swimming sperm cells and then reactivate their flagellar activity are unknown, although the ionic content of the isthmic fluid and the energy sources available to the sperm cells have been implicated in the rabbit model (Burkman *et al.*, 1984).

The events of gamete transport that immediately precede fertilization involve ovulation, tubal pickup of the oocytes and ascent of spermatozoa from the isthmic reservoir (Overstreet, 1983). The union of the gametes appears to be controlled by ovulation-associated changes in the contractility of the oviductal musculature (Battalia & Yanagimachi, 1979) and capacitation-related, intracellular changes in the spermatozoa (Cooper *et al.*, 1979). Synchronization of ovulation and sperm transport may be mediated by endocrine effects on the autonomic nervous system (Overstreet, 1983). Sperm escape from the isthmic reservoir appears to require hyperactivated flagellar activity which may also be required for fertilization (Katz *et al.*, 1989). The interrelated physiological processes in the sperm cells and the female tract are complex and it is not difficult to envisage that abnormalities in these prefertilization events could lead to subfertility. It can be speculated how prefertilization events could be influenced by DI. The previously mentioned animal studies illustrate the possibility of perturbations in gamete transport resulting from manipulations of the female tract. Current cryopreservation methods are known to alter the surfaces of spermatozoa. Thus, it is likely that the events of sperm–oviductal interaction which follow DI are different from those which occur after normal coitus. The high rates of pregnancy achieved with assisted reproductive technologies such as gamete intrafallopian transfer (GIFT) serve as important reminders that human fertilization *in vivo* can be achieved even when the normal biological processes are circumvented. It may be that the success of DI is another example of such adaptability in the reproductive system.

Acknowledgement

This research was supported in part by NIH grant HD25907.

References

Barratt, C. L. R., Chauhan, M. & Cooke, I. D. (1990). Donor insemination – a look to the future. *Fertility and Sterility*, **54**, 375–87.

Battalia, D. E. & Yanagimachi, R. (1979). Enhanced and coordinated movement of the hamster oviduct during the periovulatory period. *Journal of Reproduction and Fertility*, **56**, 515–20.

Bedford, J. M. (1970). Sperm capacitation and fertilization in mammals. *Biology of Reproduction* (Suppl.), **2**, 128–58.

Bedford, J.M. (1983). Significance of the need for sperm capacitation before fertilization in eutherian mammals. *Biology of Reproduction*, **28**, 108–20.

Brown, C. A., Boone, W. R. & Shapiro, S. S. (1988). Improved cryopreserved semen fecundability in an alternating fresh-frozen artificial insemination program. *Fertility and Sterility*, **50**, 825–7.

Burkman, L.J. (1984). Characterization of hyperactivated motility by human spermatoza during capacitation: comparison of fertile and oligospermic sperm populations. *Archives of Andrology*, **13**, 153–65.

Burkman, L. J., Overstreet, J. W. & Katz, D. F. (1984). A possible role for potassium and pyruvate in the modulation of sperm motility in the rabbit oviductal isthmus. *Journal of Reproduction and Fertility*, **71**, 367–74.

Bryd, W., Bradshaw, K., Carr, B., Edman, C., Odom, J. & Ackerman, G. (1990). A prospective randomized study of pregnancy rates following intrauterine and intracervical insemination using frozen donor sperm. *Fertility and Sterility*, **53**, 521–7.

Clisham, P. R., Drobnis, E. Z., Morales, P. M., Zinaman, M., Hanson, F. W. & Overstreet, J. W. (1989*b*). Physiology of cryopreserved sperm in the human cervix. *Journal of Andrology*, **10**, 22-P.

Clisham, P. R., Hanson, F. W., Happ, R. L., Boyers, S. P. & Overstreet, J. W. (1989*a*). Retrograde sperm migration and prolonged sperm survival in cervical mucus (CM) are common sequelae of intrauterine insemination (IUI). *Society for Gynecological Investigation*, (Abstr. 125k).

Cooper, G. W., Overstreet, J. W. & Katz, D. F. (1979). The motility of rabbit spermatozoa recovered from the female reproductive tract. *Gamete Research*, **2**, 35–42.

Corson, G. H. & Kemmann, E. (1991). The role of superovulation with menotropins in ovulatory infertility. *Fertility and Sterility*, **55**, 468–77.

Critser, J. K., Huse-Benda, A. R., Aaker, D. V., Arneson, B. W. & Ball, G. D. (1987). Cryopreservation of human spermatozoa. I. Effects of holding procedure and seeding on motility, fertilizability, and acrosome reaction. *Fertility and Sterility*, **47**, 656–63.

Cross, N. L., Morales, P., Overstreet, J. W. & Hanson, F. W. (1988). Induction of acrosome reactions by the human zona pellucida. *Biology of Reproduction*, **38**, 235–44.

Dodson, W. C. & Haney, A. F. (1991). Controlled ovarian hyperstimulation and intrauterine insemination for treatment of infertility. *Fertility and Sterility*, **55**, 457–67.

Drobnis, E. Z. & Katz, D. F. (1991). Videomicroscopy of mammalian fertilization. In *The Biology and Chemistry of Mammalian Fertilization*, P. M. Wassarman ed., pp. 269–300. New York: CRC Press, Inc.

Drobnis, E. Z., Clisham, P. R., Brazil, C. K., Hanson, F. W., Wisner, L. W. & Overstreet, J. W. (1990). An *in vitro* method of evaluating the ability of cryopreserved sperm to maintain normal physiology during residence in the female reproductive tract. *Journal of Andrology*, **11**, 53-P.

Feneux, D., Serres, C. & Jouannet, P. (1985). Sliding spermatozoa: a dyskinesia responsible for human infertility? *Fertility and Sterility*, **44**, 508–11.

Fjallbrant, B. & Ackerman, D. R. (1969). Cervical mucus penetration in vitro by fresh and frozen-preserved human semen specimens. *Journal of Reproduction and Fertility*, **20**, 515–17.

Fox, C. A., Wolff, J. S. & Baker, J. A. (1970). Measurement of intravaginal and intrauterine pressure during human coitus by radiotelemetry. *Journal of Reproduction and Fertility*, **22**, 243–51.

Gould, J. E., Overstreet, J. W. & Hanson, F. W. (1984). Assessment of human sperm function after recovery from the female reproductive tract. *Biology of Reproduction*, **31**, 888–94.

Gwatkin, R. B. L. & Anderson, O. F. (1969). Capacitation of hamster spermatozoa by bovine follicular fluid. *Nature*, **224**, 1111–12.

Hammerstedt, R. H., Graham, J. K. & Nolan, J. P. (1990). Cryopreservation of mammalian sperm: what we ask them to survive. *Journal of Andrology*, **11**, 73–88.

Hanson, F. W. & Overstreet, J. W. (1981). The interaction of human spermatozoa with cervical mucus *in vitro*. *American Journal of Obstetrics and Gynecology*, **140**, 173–8.

Hanson, F. W., Overstreet, J. W. & Katz, D. F. (1982). A study of the relationship of motile sperm numbers in cervical mucus 48 hours after artificial insemination with subsequent fertility. *American Journal of Obstetrics and Gynecology*, **143**, 89–90.

Hawk, H. W. (1987). Transport and fate of spermatozoa after insemination of cattle. *Journal of Dairy Science*, **70**, 1487–502.

Hunter, R. H. F. (1987). Human fertilization *in vivo*, with special reference to progression, storage and release of competent spermatozoa. *Human Reproduction*, **2**, 329–32.

Insler, V., Glezerman, M., Zeidel, L., Bernstein, D., Misgav, N. (1980). Sperm storage in the human cervix: a quantitative study. *Fertility and Sterility*, **23**: 288–93.

Jansen, R. P. S. (1980). Cyclic changes in the human fallopian tube isthmus and their functional importance. *American Journal of Obstetrics and Gynecology*, **201**, 349–51.

Jaszczak, S. & Hafez, E. S. E. (1973). Sperm migration through the uterine cervix in the macaque during the menstrual cycle. *American Journal of Obstetrics and Gynecology*, **115**, 1070–82.

Katz, D. F. & Drobnis, E. Z. (1990). Analysis and interpretation of the forces generated by spermatozoa. In *Fertilization in Mammals*, B. D. Bavister, J. Cummins & E. R. S. Roldan, eds, pp. 125–37. Norwell, Massachusetts: Serono Symposia, USA.

Katz, D. F., Drobnis, E. Z. & Overstreet, J. W. (1989). Factors regulating mammalian sperm migration through the female reproductive tract and oocyte vestments. *Gamete Research*, **22**, 443–69.

Katz, D.F., Morales, P., Samuels, S.J. & Overstreet, J. W. (1990). Mechanisms of filtration of morphologically abnormal human sperm by cervical mucus. *Fertility and Sterility*, **54**, 513–16.

Lambert, H., Overstreet, J. W., Morales, P., Hanson, F. W. & Yanagimachi, R. (1985). Sperm capacitation in the human female reproductive tract. *Fertility and Sterility*, **43**, 325–7.

Lightfoot, R. J. & Restall, B. J. (1971). Effects on site of insemination, sperm motility and genital tract contractions on transport of spermatozoa in the ewe. *Journal of Reproduction and Fertility*, **26**, 1–13.

Mahadevan, M. M., Trounson, A. O., Milne, B. J. & Leeton, J. F. (1982). Effect of factors related to the recipient and insemination characteristics on the success of artificial insemination with frozen semen. *Clinical Reproduction and Fertility*, **1**, 195–204.

Mattner, P. E. (1966). Formation and retention of the spermatozoon reservoir in the cervix of the ruminant. *Nature*, **212**, 1479–80.

Mattner, P. E. (1968). The distribution of spermatozoa and leucocytes in the female genital tract in goats and cattle. *Journal of Reproduction and Fertility*, **17**, 253–61.

Mazur, P. (1984). Freezing of living cells: mechanisms and implications. *American Journal of Physiology*, **247**, C125–42.

Meizel, S. (1985). Molecules that initiate or help stimulate the acrosome reaction by their interaction with the mammalian sperm surface. *American Journal of Anatomy*, **174**, 285–302.

Millet, D. & Jondet, M. (1980). Artificial insemination with frozen donor semen: Results in 604 women. In *Human Artificial Insemination and Semen Preservation*, G. David and W. S. Price, eds, pp. 259–266. New York: Plenum Press.

Moore, H. D. M. & Bedford, J. M. (1983). The interaction of mammalian gametes in the female. In *Mechanism and Control of Animal Fertilization*, J. F. Hartmann, ed. pp. 453–97. New York: Academic Press, Inc.

Morales, P., Overstreet, J. W. & Katz, D. F. (1988). Changes in human sperm movement during capacitation *in vitro*. *Journal of Reproduction and Fertility*, **83**, 119–28.

Mullins, K. J. & Saacke, R. G. (1989). Study of the functional anatomy of bovine cervical mucosa with special reference to mucus secretion and sperm transport. *Anatomical Record*, **225**, 106–17.

Overstreet, J. W. (1983). Transport of gametes in the reproductive tract of the female mammal. In *Mechanism and Control of Animal Fertilization*, J. F. Hartmann, ed., pp. 499–543. New York: Academic Press, Inc.

Overstreet, J. W. & Bedford, J. M. (1976). Embryonic mortality in the rabbit is not increased after fertilization by young epididymal spermatozoa. *Biology of Reproduction*, **15**, 54–7.

Overstreet, J. W. & Cooper, G. W. (1978). Sperm transport in the reproductive tract of the female rabbit. I. The rapid transit phase of transport. *Biology of Reproduction*, **19**, 101–14.

Overstreet, J. W. & Davis, R. O. (1992). The interaction of human spermatozoa with the fluids of the female genital tract. In *Comparative Spermatology 20 Years After*, B. Baccetti, ed., pp. 1053–8. New York: Raven Press.

Overstreet, J. W. & Katz, D. F. (1990). Interaction between the female reproductive tract and spermatozoa. In *Controls of Sperm Motility*, C. Gagnon, ed., pp. 63–75, CRC Press Inc., Boca Raton, FL.

Overstreet, J. W. & Tom, R. A. (1982). Experimental studies of rapid sperm transport in rabbits. *Journal of Reproduction and Fertility*, **66**, 601–6.

Overstreet, J. W. & VandeVoort, C. A. (1990). Sperm transport in the female
    genital tract. In *Gamete Physiology*, R. H. Asch, J. P. Balmaceda, & I.
    Johnston, eds, pp. 43–52, Norwell, MA: Serono Symposia.
Overstreet, J. W., Cooper, G. W. & Katz, D. F. (1978). Sperm transport in
    the reproductive tract of the female rabbit: II. The sustained phase of
    transport. *Biology of Reproduction*, **19**, 115–32.
Overstreet, J. W., Katz, D. F. & Cross, N. L. (1988). Sperm transport and
    capacitation. In *Gynecology and Obstetrics, Vol. V, Reproductive
    Endocrinology, Infertility and Genetics*, L. Speroff & J. L. Simpson, eds,
    Chapter 45, pp. 1–11, Philadelphia, PA: Harper and Row Publishers.
Overstreet, J. W., Katz, D. F. & Yudin, A. (1991). Cervical mucus and sperm
    transport in reproduction. *Seminars in Perinatology*,**15**, 149–55.
Robertson, L., Wolf, D. P. & Tash, J. S. (1988). Temporal changes in motility
    parameters related to acrosomal status: identification and characterization
    of populations of hyperactivated human sperm. *Biology of Reproduction*,
    39, 787–805.
Settlage, D. S. F., Motoshima, M. & Tredway, D. R. (1973). Sperm transport
    from the external cervical os to the fallopian tubes in women: a time and
    quantitation study. *Fertility and Sterility*, **24**, 655–61.
Smith, K. D., Rodriguez-Rigau, L. J. & Steinberger, E. (1981). The influence
    of ovulatory dysfunction and timing of insemination on the success of
    artificial insemination donor (AID) with fresh or cryopreserved semen.
    Fertility and Sterility, **36**, 496–502.
Smith, T. T., Koyanagi, F. & Yanagimachi, R. (1988). Quantitative
    comparison of the passage of homologous and heterologous spermatozoa
    through the uterotubal junction of the golden hamster. *Gamete Research*,
    19, 227–34.
Sobrero, A. J. & McLeod, J. (1962). The immediate post-coital test. *Fertility
    and Sterility*, **13**, 184–9.
Suarez, S. S. (1987). Sperm transport and motility in the mouse oviduct:
    observations *in situ*. *Biology of Reproduction*, **36**, 203–10.
Suarez, S. S., Wolf, D. P. & Meizel, S. (1986). Induction of the acrosome
    reaction in human spermatozoa by a fraction of human follicular fluid.
    Gamete Research, **14**, 107–21.
Tredway, D. R., Buchanan, G. C. & Drake, T. S. (1978). Comparison of the
    fractional post-coital test and semen analysis. *American Journal of
    Obstetrics and Gynecology*, **130**, 647–52.
Ulstein, M. (1973). Fertility, motility and penetration in cervical mucus of
    freeze-preserved human spermatozoa. *Acta Obstetricia and Gynecologica
    Scandinavica*, **52**, 205–10.
Watson, P. F. (1985). Recent advances in sperm freezing. In *In Vitro
    Fertilization and Donor Insemination*, W. Thompson, D. N. Joyce and J.
    R. Newton, eds, pp. 261–7. New York: Perinatology Press.
Yanagimachi, R. (1969). *In vitro* acrosome reaction and capacitation of golden
    hamster spermatozoa by bovine follicular fluid and its fractions. *Journal of
    Experimental Zoology*, **170**, 269–80.
Yanagimachi, R. (1981). Mechanisms of fertilization in mammals. In
    Fertilization and Embryonic Development In Vitro, L. Mastroianni and J.
    D. Biggers, eds, pp. 81–182. New York: Plenum Press.
Yanagimachi, R. (1988). Mammalian fertilization. In *The Physiology of
    Reproduction*, E. Knobil & J. Neill *et al.*, eds. pp. 135–85. New York:
    Raven Press, Ltd.

Yudin, A. I., Hanson, F. W. & Katz, D. F. (1989). Human cervical mucus and its interaction with sperm: a fine-structural view. *Biology of Reproduction*, **40**, 661–71.

Zavos, P. M., & Cohen, M. R. (1980). Bovine mucus penetration test: an assay for fresh and cryopreserved human spermatozoa. *Fertility and Sterility*, **34**, 175–6.

Zinaman, M., Drobnis, E. Z., Morales, P., Brazil, C. K., Kiel, M., Cross, N. L., Hanson, F. W. & Overstreet, J. W. (1989). The physiology of sperm recovered from the human cervix: acrosomal status and response to inducers of the acrosome reaction. *Biology of Reproduction*, **41**, 790–7.

5

Techniques for examining the fertilizing capacity of semen

D. W. RICHARDSON and R. J. AITKEN

Introduction

A prerequisite for a successful donor insemination programme is the employment of objective methods for the evaluation of semen in order to facilitate the selection of optimal specimens for cryostorage and subsequent insemination. During the past decade, the descriptive criteria that comprise the conventional semen analysis have been supplemented by a second generation of tests, focussing on the functional competence of spermatozoa rather than their appearance. These functional tests have included:

1. assessment of the acrosome reaction using labelled lectins and monoclonal antibodies using reagents such as A23187 to activate these cells (Cross *et al.*, 1986: Aitken, 1988);
2. the hamster oocyte penetration test, for which there is data from prospective studies indicating a significant relationship with male fertility (Aitken, Irvine & Wu, 1991);
3. the hypo-osmotic swelling (HOS) test, which has been advocated as a means of evaluating the functional integrity of the sperm plasma membrane (Jeyendran *et al.*, 1984);
4. the detailed analysis of the movement characteristics of spermatozoa, using video- and time lapse exposure-photomicrography (Overstreet *et al.*, 1979; Mathur *et al.*, 1986);
5. the sperm–mucus penetration test (SMP) which has been claimed to show a close relationship with other aspects of human sperm function including their movement (Aitken, Warner & Reid, 1986) and their capacity for sperm–oocyte fusion (Aitken *et al.*, 1985);

6. measurement of a variety of biochemical parameters such as ATP (Comhaire *et al.*, 1983), creatine phosphokinase (Huszar & Vigue, 1990) and reactive oxygen species generation (Aitken & Clarkson, 1987), which correlate, to varying extents, with the fertilizing ability of human spermatozoa.

In this chapter, the principles behind each of these criteria of semen quality will be reviewed and their clinical significance assessed with particular emphasis on the evaluation of donors for artificial insemination programmes. However, before embarking on a discussion of these functional assays, the relative merits of the conventional semen profile will be considered.

Conventional criteria of semen quality

The conventional semen analysis provides descriptive information on 1) semen volume, 2) the concentration of spermatozoa and their total number in the ejaculate, 3) sperm agglutination, 4) motility and 5) sperm morphology, together with an assessment of semen liquefaction and viscosity. In addition, pH can be measured, as can biochemical indicators of seminal vesicle and prostate function, in order to provide clinically relevant information about the normality of spermatogenesis and the patency of the reproductive tract (World Health Organization, 1987).

Although these criteria provide a profile of the semen and furnish data for the clinical andrologist, they only provide a superficial descriptive analysis of the numbers of motile and structurally normal spermatozoa in the semen. They give little indication regarding the functional competence and fertilizing potential of the spermatozoa, which is clearly the key question to be addressed when selecting donors for artificial insemination.

The limitations of the conventional semen profile as a means of assessing male fertility have been repeatedly analysed (Barratt *et al.*, 1989; De Kretser, Yates & Kovacs, 1985; Van Uem *et al.*, 1985; Hirsch *et al.*, 1986; Hewitt, Cohen & Steptoe, 1987). For example, Polansky and Lamb (1988), in their prospective study involving 1089 couples attending an infertility clinic, found no significant influence of any semen characteristic on the cumulative probability of conception, and were sceptical of the usefulness of such criteria in predicting the future fertility of infertile couples. Similarly, Aiman (1982) found no relationship between either sperm concentration or motility and conception *in vivo* in 81 women receiving donor insemination for a maximum of six cycles of insemination.

The subjectivity inherent in certain aspects of the conventional semen profile such as morphology, is one of the reasons underlying its inadequacy. The failure to use standardized, universally accepted methods of evaluation is another, despite the efforts of the World Health Organization to address this problem. Inadequate training of laboratory technicians in the procedures used to construct a semen profile may also have a considerable impact on the results obtained. Hence, in relation to inaccuracies in the measurement of sperm density, an overall coefficient of variation of the order of 5% was reported by Freund and Carol (1964), whereas Jequier and Ukombe (1983) found coefficients of variation of 44.3%, and 8.2% to 32.8% respectively for between-technician and within-technician determinations.

Significant observer-dependent variability in motility determinations has also been reported, with Jequier and Ukombe (1983) finding a 30%–80% variation between 26 observers, whilst an inter-technician coefficient of variation of 10.4 to 15.5 was calculated by Zaini, Jennings and Baker (1985). In terms of sperm morphology, Ayodeji and Baker (1986), reported statistically significant differences in the assessment of sperm morphology on an inter- and intra-technician basis, emphasizing the limited value of this criterion of semen quality (Baker & Clarke, 1987). These conclusions echo the results obtained 20 years earlier by Freund (1966) in a multi-centre survey involving a comparative study of sperm morphology in which 47 laboratories participated. He concluded that the criteria applied by different observers were qualitative, personally orientated, subjective and non-repeatable. These comments could probably have been generally applied to results emanating from several laboratories for the next decade and have led to a general call for the introduction of standardized techniques of laboratory semen analysis from several authorities including Freund (1962, 1966), Freund and Carol (1964), Eliasson (1971, 1973, 1975, 1981), Freund and Peterson (1976).

The requirement for standardized methodology in semen analysis had been recognized by the World Heath Organization with the publication of their laboratory manuals for the examination of human semen (World Health Organization, 1980, 1987). Adoption of the WHO protocols should ultimately improve standards of semen analysis and decrease inter-laboratory variability in results.

The successful use of standardized techniques to reduce variability resulting from technician error, was reported by Mortimer, Shu and Tan

(1986) who, after training technicians to a high standard, achieved very high correlations between sperm concentration determinations and a 96.6% agreement regarding motility. Similarly, Dunphy *et al.* (1989) reported non-significant inter-technician error in determinations of sperm concentration, and both they and Overstreet and Katz (1987) again stressed the necessity of standardization of all facets of seminal analysis and of systematic quality control.

There can be no doubt that the overall standards of practice in seminology laboratories could be significantly improved if standardized protocols were followed, and thorough training of technicians provided at workshops organized under the auspices of a recognized professional society.

Sperm function tests applicable to donor insemination

The conventional semen analysis provides basic data relating to sperm numbers, motility and morphology. However, irrespective of the degree of technological refinement, the traditional spermiogram will remain inadequate because the information it provides is essentially descriptive. It does not give precise diagnostic information concerning the functional competence of the spermatozoa and has been shown to be of limited prognostic value in prospective studies (Aitken, Irvine & Wu, 1991). These limitations of the standard semen analysis have acted as an impetus for the development of additional tests to supplement the data provided by the routine spermiogram.

It is important that the selection of semen for therapeutic donor insemination (DI) is highly efficient, because only 10–20% of men tested as potential donors for DI programmes are finally accepted (Chauhan *et al.*, 1988). The reasons for the high exclusion rate include (1) an abnormal semen profile, (2) semen being consistently of a low volume, (3) aspects of the potential donor's, or his family's medical history being unacceptable, (4) the susceptibility of the semen to cryopreservation and (5) a failure to establish pregnancies. It is also imperative that only the most fertile samples are employed for DI because, inevitably, a considerable amount of time and effort is invested in the recruitment, counselling and screening of donors before they are finally accepted into such programmes.

Many authors support the contention that sperm function tests are superior to traditional semen parameters in the prediction of the fertilizing capacity of spermatozoa including Irvine (1986), Aitken *et al.* (1988),

Lui *et al.* (1988), Aitken (1989), Barratt *et al.* (1989), Holt *et al.* (1989) and Barratt, Chauhan and Cooke (1990). In the context of donor insemination, the tests that are currently available should provide data on the ability of donor spermatozoa to: (1) penetrate and traverse the cervical mucus (2) ascend the female reproductive tract (3) undergo capacitation and the acrosome reaction (4) generate the fusogenic equatorial segment (5) penetrate the zona pellucida then (6) undergo nuclear decondensation. All these events, apart from possibly (2) can be evaluated by laboratory tests of sperm function.

The acrosome reaction

An important physiological event that spermatozoa must undergo during the fertilization of the ovum is the completion of the acrosome reaction so that, in theory, evaluation of this event should provide information relevant to the potential fertility of the spermatozoa. To assess the completion of the acrosome reaction, tests have been developed that utilize monoclonal antibodies or lectins targeted against specific constituents of the acrosome, enabling loss of the acrosomal contents or outer acrosomal membrane to be monitored. In interpreting information obtained in this way, it is important to be able to distinguish the normal physiological acrosome reaction from pathological acrosomal loss, secondary to a loss of viability. This problem has been overcome by incorporating into the protocols used to detect the acrosome reaction, supra-vital stains, such as Hoechst 33258 (Cross *et al.*, 1986) which exhibit a limited ability to penetrate viable cells. Consequently, spermatozoa which demonstrate reduced monoclonal antibody binding over the acrosomal region, together with an absence of vital staining, are considered to have undergone a normal acrosome reaction (Cross *et al.*, 1986).

Despite the development of such tests, the acrosome reaction is unlikely to be employed as a routine criterion of potential sperm function because: (1) very low rates of acrosome reaction are observed with human sperm populations incubated *in vitro*, even when such incubations are prolonged for 24 hours, and 2) the natural stimulus for the acrosome reaction is thought to be a glycoprotein component of the human zona pellucida ZP3, which cannot be isolated in sufficient quantities to test the fuctional properties of human spermatozoa on a routine, diagnostic basis. Since alternative reagents for inducing the acrosome reaction, such as A23187, are of limited efficiency in populations of human spermatozoa, this criterion of human sperm function may not be of significant value until a biologically active form of recombinant human ZP3 becomes available.

The hamster oocyte penetration test (HPT)

This test generates information on a number of the critical physiological events essential for fertilization. It furnishes information upon (a) sperm capacitation and the acrosome reaction (b) the ability of spermatozoa to generate a fusogenic equatorial segment and to fuse with the vitelline membrane of the oocyte, and (c) sperm nuclear decondensation. The hamster egg penetration test is based upon the original report of inter-species fertilization by Yanagimachi (1972) who demonstrated that guinea pig spermatozoa could penetrate zona-free hamster oocytes. This observation was followed by the significant finding that acrosome reacted human spermatozoa could also penetrate such oocytes by Yana-gimachi, Yanagimachi and Rogers (1976). The basic methodology has been modified in many different ways since the original description (Barros *et al.*, 1979; Rogers *et al.*, 1979, 1983; Aitken, 1985; Aitken *et al.*, 1982*a*, 1982*b*, 1983, 1984*b*, 1985; Aitken & Elton, 1984, 1986) with the result that the evaluation of this test has suffered from a lack of standardization. The standardized protocol recommended by the World Health Organization (1987) involves a 24 hour pre-incubation period in a simple, defined culture medium, in order to capacitate the cells, prior to the introduction of the zona-free oocytes (Aitken, 1985). An important modification, which reduces variability due to differences between individuals in the rate of sperm capacitation, has been to include the calcium ionophore A23187 in the sperm suspension. Its inclusion increases the levels of free intracellular calcium and accelerates and synchronizes the induction of the acrosome reaction, enhancing the incidence of sperm-oocyte fusion, and thereby increasing the sensitivity of the assay (Aitken *et al.*, 1984*a*).

In retrospective studies involving patients exhibiting varicoele, asthenozoospermia or oligozoospermia, hamster oocyte fusion rates have been recorded which are consistently below the normal fertile range (Aitken *et al.*, 1982*b*, 1984*b*, 1985; Rogers, 1985; Aitken & Elton 1986; Plymate *et al.*, 1987). In a prospective study involving patients with unexplained infertility, it was reported that conception rates exhibited a linear increase in concert with hamster oocyte penetration scores in the range from 0 to 75%, in an HPT protocol lacking A23187. When the results of the HPT were considered in conjunction with data from the traditional spermiogram and sperm movement characteristics, a combination of variables could be identified which, when subjected to a multivariate discriminant analysis, achieved a prediction of fertility which was 85% accurate (Aitken *et al.*, 1984*b*).

If a comparable analysis were to be applied in the selection of prospective donor semen for donor insemination, it should markedly increase the potential success of such semen in achieving conception. A relevant study was reported by Irvine and Aitken (1986), when they evaluated the predictive value of 25 variables applied to cryostored semen, used in donor insemination treatment. They subjected each sample to an analysis comprising the conventional semen profile, sperm movement characteristics, ATP measurements of spermatozoa and semen, and the HPT performed in the presence of A21387. A sample was considered successful if it produced a pregnancy within a minimum of four cycles of insemination. In this study, 3 of the 25 variables used in the analysis showed statistically significant differences between successful and unsuccessful ejaculates: (1) the concentration of motile spermatozoa in the insemination sample, (2) the percentage of motile sperm following A23187 incubation, and (3) the mean number of spermatozoa penetrating each oocyte in the A23187-enhanced HPT, were incorporated in a multivariate discriminant analysis. On the basis of the HPT results alone, a prediction of the ability of individual cryostored samples to establish pregnancies *in vivo* could be obtained which was about 75% accurate. If these data were combined with information describing the movement characteristics of the spermatozoa, the accuracy of this prediction could be increased to about 85%.

The diagnostic value of the A23187-enchanced HPT has been further supported by the results of a recent prospective trial involving 139 couples, characterized by a lack of detectable abnormalities in the female partner and followed up for a maximum of 4 years. During this time, 32 patients (23%) conceived in the absence of therapeutic intervention. Life table analysis indicated the existence of a significant relationship between the outcome of the A23187-enhanced HPT and fertility, such that patients exhibiting less than 10% oocyte penetration were five times less likely to establish a pregnancy than those exhibiting HPT scores above this arbitrary threshold (Aitken *et al.*, 1991). Furthermore, a false negative rate of only 4% was observed in this data set, since only 1 out of

24 patients exhibiting a 0% HPT result, spontaneously initiated a pregnancy during the follow-up period. This low incidence of false negative scores is extremely important, because it is these results, purporting to indicate the complete absence of fertilizing potential, that bear heavily on patient management and, in a DI context, would have the greatest impact on donor selection. The significance of these results is underlined by the fact that within the same prospective data base, the conventional criteria of semen quality were found to be of no prognostic value whatsoever.

The hamster oocyte penetration test is, therefore, clinically useful and measures several key components of normal sperm function. However, interpretation of the results obtained with this test should be tempered by an awareness that it is not a global test of human sperm function in that there are several aspects of sperm cell biology that it does not address. This applies particularly to aspects of human sperm function involving sperm movement, since, even completely immotile spermatozoa, for example, those exhibiting Kartagener's syndrome, can initiate fusion with the vitelline membrane of the zona-free hamster oocyte (Aitken, Ross and Lees, 1983). The HPT should therefore be used in conjunction with other tests that analyse additional aspects of sperm function, particularly those dependent on sperm movement. In this way, an integrated group of tests might be developed to give as accurate an assessment of the fertilizing potential of donor semen as possible.

Hypo-osmotic swelling test

The proponents of this test (HOS) suggest that it measures the functional integrity of the sperm plasma membrane. It is based on the premise that when spermatozoa are incubated in a hypo-osmotic medium, then, provided the plasma membrane is intact, water will enter the cells in order to achieve an osmotic equilibrium. This influx of water causes the spermatozoa to swell and, providing the plasma membrane has sufficient elasticity to accommodate this influx, there will be a sudden increase in intracellular volume, manifested by a coiling of the sperm tail. Scoring of the HOS test is based on the percentage of spermatozoa that show coiled tails and the results can be taken to reflect the properties of the sperm plasma membrane in terms of its integrity and viscoelasticity.

It was claimed by Jeyendran *et al.* (1984) that the HOS test provided a better predictive indicator than conventional semen parameters in the prediction of successful HPT results, although his conclusion was based

on only 23 semen specimens. Van der Ven *et al.* (1986) also concluded
that the HOS test gave a more accurate prediction of successful *in vitro*
fertilization than did traditional semen parameters, but, because of the
number of false positive and negative results, it was suggested that the
HOS test required more extensive trials.

After rigorous evaluation, a number of authors have concluded that
the HOS test does not offer satisfactory predictability relative to HPT or
IVF results. Hence Chan *et al.* (1985) in a study involving 270 semen
specimens from fertile and infertile men, found no significant correlation
between the HOS test and the HPT results. Similarly, Lui *et al.* (1988)
and Barratt *et al.* (1989) concluded that the outcome of the HOS was of no
predictive value in terms of IVF success.

It is perhaps too simplistic to expect that a single test based on the
physical integrity of the spermatozoon will be able to assess the multi-
plicity of functions associated with the sperm plasma membrane and, in
clinical terms, there appears to be a consensus that the HOS test is of little
diagnostic value.

Sperm movement

Several of the most critical events in conception are dependent upon
sperm motility, including penetration of the cervical mucus and penetration through the outer investments of the ovum, particularly the zona
pellucida.

The traditional semen analysis provides information relating to the
percentage of sperm showing motility, together with a subjective assessment of progressiveness but does not include an objective evaluation of
the quality of sperm movement. During the past decade, there has been
rapid progress towards the development of objective methods to quanti-
tate the movement characteristics of human spermatozoa. These
methods have been based on ultra-violet and laser light scattering (Lee *et
al.*, 1982; Mayevsky, Dafna & Bastov, 1980), videomicrography (Katz &
Overstreet, 1980), cinemicrography (David, Serres & Jouannet, 1981)
and time-exposure photomicrography (Overstreet *et al.*, 1979, Milligan,
Harris & Dennis, 1980; Aitken *et al.*, 1982*a,c*).

The ultra-violet and laser-light scattering methods provide objective
data concerning the overall degree of movement in semen and also have
the advantage of sampling a large number of cells. However these
methods fail to furnish any data on the individual components of sperm
movement.

The most detailed evaluation of the components of sperm movement is achieved using cinemicrography, which resolves both head and flagellar activity. Unfortunately, this technique samples a low number of spermatozoa and is very labour-intensive. The time-exposure photomicrography method is simple to perform and provides data on linear velocity of sperm progression, amplitude of lateral head displacement and the frequency of head rotation – all attributes of movement with functional significance. However, this method is also labour intensive and samples a limited number of cells.

Computerized videomicrography (Mathur *et al.*, 1986) is expensive, but provides a realistic combination of resolution and sample size and has considerable potential in the future. A detailed survey of the equipment and techniques available for the analysis of semen, including the automatic quantitative determination of sperm movement, is outside the remit of this chapter. However, Mortimer (1990) has recently reviewed this topic.

The clinical study of the various computerized systems that are currently available for assessing sperm movement is largely contingent upon the existence of data indicating that there is, in fact, a close relationship between the movement characteristics of human spermatozoa and fertility. In this context, the significance of the velocity of linear progression (V_p) was shown to be a major discriminating variable, positively related to the fertilizing capacity of human ejaculates in a DI clinic (Irvine & Aitken, 1986; Holt *et al.*, 1989). This finding is in agreement with the results obtained by Holt, Moore and Hillier (1985), who, using a semi-automatic computerized technique, showed that V_p correlated significantly with both HPT and human IVF results. In addition, they concluded that these velocity measurements, when incorporated into a multivariate discriminant analysis, could be used to predict the results of such *in vitro* tests with almost 75% accuracy.

A second important movement characteristic is the amplitude of lateral head displacement, which is directly related to successful penetration of the investments surrounding the egg, particularly the zona pellucida (Jeulin *et al.*, 1986; Katz, Drobnis & Overstreet (1989) and also plays a critical role in the successful penetration of cervical mucus by human spermatozoa (Aitken *et al.*, 1985; Aitken, Warner & Reid, 1986). In their analysis of DI donors, Irvine and Aitken (1986) showed that a low amplitude of lateral head displacement was strongly negatively related to fertility and that this criterion, in combination with other aspects of sperm movement, could predict the fertility of DI donors with 73% accuracy.

Cervical mucus penetration

A variety of factors influence the passage of spermatozoa through cervical mucus, including the physico-chemical state of the mucus and the activity of seminal enzymes, which act to lyse the sub-structure of the mucus and thereby enhance the progress of the spermatozoa through this barrier. Another crucial element which governs the penetration of spermatozoa through the mucus, is their intrinsic motility and in particular, the quality of their movement.

Assessment of the ability of spermatozoa to penetrate cervical mucus has been the focus of a variety of test methods but the most widely accepted protocols have been modifications of the Kremer test (Kremer, 1965). One example of such a test was the method developed by Katz, Overstreet and Hanson (1980) to yield a PSC value (percentage successful collisions). This system provides a quantitative index of successful cervical mucus penetration, calculated from the number of spermatozoa which penetrated the cervical mucus during a 30-minute incubation period and the number and velocity of spermatozoa in the original semen specimen. The PSC result is taken to indicate the percentage of sperm collisions with the cervical mucus interface which culminate in successful mucus penetration.

In studies involving the application of PSC analysis, Aitken *et al.* (1985, 1986) showed that 76% of the variation in their cervical mucus penetration results could be accounted for by differences in the patterns of sperm motility. In these studies, the most important characteristic of sperm movement in relation to cervical mucus penetration was the degree of lateral sperm head displacement. They reported a negative correlation between the proportion of spermatozoa showing a low degree of lateral sperm head displacement and cervical mucus penetration and, conversely, a strong positive correlation between the absolute amplitude of lateral head displacement and successful penetration of cervical mucus. Lateral head displacement is of significance because it reflects the amplitude of the flagellar beating envelope (David *et al.*, 1981) and it is the amplitude of the flagellar wave that governs the foward thrust developed by the spermatozoa when immobilized at a surface, such as the cervical mucus interface. Larger amplitudes of lateral head displacement result in greater forward thrust and help drive the sperm head across the interface into the cervical mucus.

The inability of spermatozoa displaying small amplitudes of lateral head displacement to penetrate cervical mucus was emphasized by the results of Feneux, Serres & Jouannet (1985) and Aitken *et al.* (1986). Mortimer, Pandya and Sawers (1986), using a scoring system different to the PSC method, reached similar conclusions. They found the concentration of motile spermatozoa, the mean amplitude of lateral head displacement, mean progressive velocity and the percentage of morphologically normal spermatozoa to be the most significant variables, and entry of these variables into a discriminant equation, provided a prediction that was 75.4% accurate as to whether cervical mucus penetration was abnormal or normal.

Barratt *et al.* (1989), using the sperm mucus penetration (SMP) test described by Pandya *et al.* (1986), found that this system was an effective discriminator of the fertilizing capacity of human spermatozoa *in vitro*, and no false negatives were recorded. They considered the SMP test warranted further investigation as a criterion of human sperm quality and suggested it could be used in combination with other functional tests in the analysis of male infertility.

Biochemical tests of sperm function

Although bioassays of sperm function, such as the HPT, generate valuable data relating to fertility, they are highly labour intensive and require specialized knowledge as well as animal facilities. Consequently, in the next decade, the emphasis will be on developing a series of alternative, biochemical tests, which also provide information on the potential fertility of spermatozoa but which can be readily standardized and performed in non-specialized laboratories.

Measurement of ATP

It has been proposed that the measurement of ATP could provide a valid measure of the fertilizing potential of human spermatozoa (Comhaire *et al.*, 1983), and also serve as a means of assessing frozen specimens used in donor insemination, (Comhaire and Vermeulen, 1986). However, when Irvine and Aitken (1986) measured ATP concentration in cryostored ejaculates utilized in a donor insemination service and incorporated this parameter in a multivariate discriminant analysis, no discrimination of successful and unsuccessful ejaculates was possible. They considered that the ATP relationships described by Comhaire *et al*, (1983) were principally dependent upon the close correlation between motility and sperm numbers, and concluded that the measurement of ATP levels in semen did not constitute a valid biochemical marker for the prediction of fertilizing ability *in vivo*.

Chan and Wang (1987) confirmed the findings of Comhaire *et al*. (1983) in that there was a positive correlation between ATP concentration in semen and sperm motility and count, however they found no correlation between ATP concentration and sperm fertilizing capacity, in concord with Irvine and Aitken (1986). They also concluded that seminal ATP determinations did not appear to be a definitive marker of the fertilizing ability of spermatozoa.

Determination of reactive oxygen species.

An association has been observed between the excessive generation of reactive oxygen species by the washed human ejaculate and the functional competence of the spermatozoa (Aitken & Clarkson, 1987; Aitken *et al.*, 1987). This excessive generation of reactive oxygen species results in peroxidation of the unsaturated fatty acids in the sperm plasma membrane and, by reducing membrane fluidity, impairs the ability of affected cells to engage in the membrane fusion events associated with fertilization.

Relationships between reactive oxygen species generation and the fertilizing ability of human spermatozoa *in vivo* and *in vitro* have been established under conditions where the conventional semen profile was of no diagnostic value (Aitken, 1989; Aitken *et al*. 1991). Elevated levels of oxidant production are observed in association with the infiltration of leucocytes into the ejaculate (Aitken & West, 1990) and/or as a consequence of defects in the spermatozoa themselves, as is frequently observed in cases of oligozoospermia.

An implication of these observations is that it could be of clinical benefit to determine the levels of reactive oxygen species in the semen of prospective donors. In such a screening programme, low levels of reactive oxygen species generation would be a positive indicator of potential fertility.

Post-thaw motility and cryosurvival

The value of post-thaw motility (PTM) and the consequent cryosurvival as a predictive variable in the evaluation of the fertility of donor semen has been stressed by several groups. David *et al*. (1980) reported significantly higher conception rates achieved with semen showing heightened post-thaw motilities, in that a 17% conception rate was achieved with cryostored semen showing PTMs >65%, whereas only a 7% rate of conception was recorded with semen having <40% post-thaw motilities. Mayaux *et al.* (1985) also concluded that the PTM and sperm morphology were the most important factors in predicting the fertility of donor semen. Irvine and Aitken (1986) measured the movement characteristics of cryostored human spermatozoa after they had been washed free of seminal plasma and incubated *in vitro* for 3 hours. These measurements of post thaw movement were shown to be significantly related to the fertilizing ability of the spermatozoa *in vivo* and in combination with assessments of sperm–oocyte fusion in the HPT, could predict the fertility of samples in a DI programme with more than 80% accuracy.

Applications of sperm function tests in the selection of semen for donor insemination

In view of the considerable amount of time and effort that must be expended in recruiting and screening donors for artificial insemination, it is axiomatic that only the most fertile specimens are subject to cryostorage. The data presented in this brief review indicate that a number of functional assays are now available to facilitate this selection process. A normal semen profile, constructed using the guidelines laid down by the World Health Organization (1987) and including analyses of sperm count, motility and morphology, is a fundamental requirement for any semen donor. The descriptive analysis of the semen sample should also include an assessment of leucocytic infiltration, since the presence of such cells may be indicative of a reproductive tract infection in the donor. Furthermore the release of reactive oxygen species by activated leucocytes may compromise the functional competence of the spermatozoa (Barratt, Bolton & Cooke, 1990). Although a concentration of one million leucocytes per ml has been set as the upper limit of normality by the World Health Organization (1987), there is no rational basis for this threshold and lower concentrations of these cells could be damaging, depending on their site of origin and state of activation (Aitken & West, 1990).

An accurate assessment of the fertilizing capacity of a potential donor will require that the descriptive semen profile is supplemented with additional techniques to monitor the functional competence of the spermatozoa. At the present time, the most informative method of assessing human sperm function is probably the zona-free hamster oocyte penetration test. This assay generates important data on the capacity of the spermatozoa to acrosome react and initiate fusion with the vitelline membrane of the oocyte. In order to increase the sensitivity of the technique, the ionophore A23187 should be included in the protocol to facilitate the induction of the acrosome reaction. The reliability of the assay should be assessed by including appropriate positive control samples in every test (Aitken, 1986). Performed in this manner, the HPT has been shown to predict the fertilizing potential of samples in an artificial insemination programme with considerable accuracy (Irvine & Aitken, 1986).

The major defect of the HPT is that a successful outcome does not depend on the motility of the spermatozoa. Since sperm motility is essential for fertilization to occur, measurements of the movement characteristics of these cells should be used to supplement the data obtained with the hamster oocyte assay. The recent introduction of automatic, computerized image analysis systems to monitor the move-ment characteristics of human spermatozoa has greatly facilitated the collection of such data. Moreover, a combination of data describing the movement characteristics of human spermatozoa and their capacity for sperm–oocyte fusion has been shown to predict the fertility of cryostored samples employed in a DI programme with more than 80% accuracy (Irvine & Aitken, 1986).

Future developments will focus on the use of biochemical criteria to monitor human sperm function that will be easier to standardize and perform than bioassays such as the HPT. Already a number of biochemi-cal markers are beginning to emerge, such as the measurement of reactive oxygen species. Additional criteria will be added to this list in concert with advances in our knowledge of the cell biology of the human spermatozoon and the influence of cryostorage upon its functional integrity.

It would be unrealistic to suggest that such sperm function tests could be carried out at all centres providing donor insemination. However, if, in Great Britain, eight supra-regional centres were established for the cryostorage of semen for DI, and from these principal cryo-banks, semen was distributed to requesting agencies (e.g. subfertility clinics, hospitals, clinicians, satellite centres) then virtually all donor recruitment, screen-ing and semen evaluation, including the listed tests of sperm function, could be carried out at these primary centres. If this network were to be established, then a significant improvement in both DI service, treatment and results would be expected in Britain.

References

Aiman, J. (1982). Factors affecting the success of donor insemination. *Fertility and Sterility*, **37**, 94–9.

Aitken, R. J. (1985). Diagnostic value of the zona-free hamster oocyte penetration test and sperm movement characteristics in oligozoospermia. *International Journal of Andrology*, **8**, 348–56.

Aitken, R. J. (1986). The zona-free hamster oocyte penetration test and the diagnosis of male fertility. *International Journal of Andrology*, Suppl. 6, 199.

Aitken, R. J. (1988). Assessment of sperm function for IVF. *Human Reproduction*, **3**, 89–95.

Aitken, R. J. (1989). Assessment of human sperm function. In *The Testis*, 2nd edn. H. Burger and D. de Kretser, eds, pp. 441–73, New York: Raven Press Ltd.

Aitken, R. J. (1990). Evaluation of human sperm function. *British Medical Bulletin*, **46**, 654–74

Aitken, R. J. & Clarkson, J. S. (1987). Cellular basis of defective sperm function and its association with the genesis of reactive oxygen species by human spermatozoa. *Journal of Reproduction and Fertility*, **81**, 459–69.

Aitken, R. J. & Elton, R. A. (1984). Significance of Poisson distribution theory in analysing the interaction between human spermatozoa and zona-free hamster oocytes. *Journal of Reproduction and Fertility*, **72**, 311–21.

Aitken, R. J. & Elton, R. A. (1986). Application of a Poisson-gamma model to study the influence of gamete concentration on sperm–oocyte fusion in the zona-free hamster egg penetration test. *Journal of Reproduction and Fertility*, **78**, 733–9.

Aitken, R. J. & West, K. M. (1990). Relationship between reactive oxygen species generation and leucocyte infiltration in fractions isolated from the human ejaculate on Percoll gradients. *International Journal of Andrology*, **13**, 433–51.

Aitken, R. J., Best, F. S. M., Richardson, D. W., Djahanbakhch, O. & Lees, M. M. (1982*a*). The correlates of fertilizing capacity in normal fertile men. *Fertility and Sterility*, **38**, 68–76.

Aitken, R. J., Best, F. S. M., Richardson, D. W., Djahanbakhch, O., Templeton, A. A. & Lees, M. M. (1982*b*). An analysis of semen quality and sperm function in cases of oligozoospermia. *Fertility and Sterility*, **38**, 705–11.

Aitken, R. J., Best, F. S. M., Richardson, D. W., Djahanbakhch, O., Mortimer, D., Templeton, A. A. & Lees, M. M. (1982*c*). An analysis of sperm function in cases of unexplained infertility; conventional criteria, movement characteristics and fertilizing capacity. *Fertility and Sterility*, **38**, 212–21.

Aitken, R. J., Best, F. S. M., Warner, P. & Templeton, A. A. (1984*a*). A prospective study of the relationship between semen quality and fertility in cases of unexplained infertility. *Journal of Andrology*, **5**, 297–303.

Aitken, R. J., Clarkson, J. S., Huang, G. F. & Irvine, D. S. (1987). Cell biology of defective sperm function. In *New Horizons in Sperm Cell Research*. H. Mohin, ed., pp. 75–89, New York: Gordon and Breach.

Aitken, R. J., Irvine, D. S., Clarkson, J. & Richardson, D. W. (1988). Development of in vitro systems for the diagnosis of human sperm function. In *Advances in Clinical Andrology*, C. L. R. Barratt and I. D. Cooke, eds, pp. 99–112, Lancaster, UK: MTP Press.

Aitken, R. J., Irvine, D. S. & Wu, F. C. W. (1992). Prospective analysis of sperm–oocyte fusion and reactive oxygen species generation as criteria for the diagnosis of infertility. *American Journal of Obstetrics and Gynecology* (in press).

Aitken, R. J., Ross, A., Hargreave, T., Richardson, D. & Best, F. (1984b). Analysis of human sperm function following exposure to the ionophore A23187. *Journal of Andrology*, **5**, 321–9.

Aitken, R. J., Ross, A. & Lees, M. M. (1983). Analysis of sperm function in Kartagener's syndrome. *Fertility and Sterility*, **40**, 696–8.

Aitken, R. J., Sutton, M., Warner, P. & Richardson, D. W. (1985). Relationship between the movement characteristics of human spermatozoa and their ability to penetrate cervical mucus and zona-free hamster oocytes. *Journal of Reproduction and Fertility*, **73**, 441–9.

Aitken, R. J., Wang, Y. F., Lui, J., Best, F. S. M. & Richardson, D. W. (1983). The influence of medium composition, osmolarity and albumen content on the acrosome reaction and fertilizing capacity of human spermatozoa: development of an improved zona free hamster egg penetration test. *International Journal of Andrology*, **5**, 180–93.

Aitken, R. J., Warner, P. E. & Reid, C. P. (1986). Factors influencing the success of sperm–cervical mucus interaction in patients exhibiting unexplained infertility. *Journal of Andrology*, **7**, 3–10.

Ayodeji, O. & Baker, H. W. G. (1986). Is there a specific abnormality of sperm morphology in men with varicocoeles. *Fertility and Sterility*, **45**, 839–42.

Baker, H. W. G. & Clarke, G. N. (1987). Sperm morphology: consistency of assessment of the same sperm by different observers. *Clinical Reproduction and Fertility*, **5**, 37–43.

Barratt, C. L. R., Bolton, A. E. & Cooke, I. D. (1990). Functional significance of white blood cells in the male and female reproductive tract. *Human Reproduction*, **5**, 639–48.

Barratt, C. L. R., Osborn, J. C., Harrison, P. E., Monks, N., Dunphy, B. C., Lenton, E. A. & Cooke, I. D. (1989). The hypo-osmotic swelling test and the sperm mucus penetration test in determining fertilization of the human oocyte. *Human Reproduction*, **4**, 430–4.

Barratt, C. L. R. & Chauhan, M. (1990). Human donor insemination (Review). *Bibliography of Reproduction*, **55**(1). A1–8.

Barratt, C. L. R., Chauhan, M. & Cooke, I. D. (1990). Donor insemination – a look to the future. *Fertility and Sterility*, **54**, 375–87.

Barros, C., Gonzalez, J., Herrera, E., Bustos, O. & Bregon, E. (1979). Human sperm penetration into zona-free hamster oocytes as a test to evaluate the fertilizing ability. *Andrologia*, **11**, 197–210.

Chan, S. Y. W., Fox, E. J., Chan, M. M. C., Tsoi, W., Wang, C., Tang, L. C. H., Tang, G. W. K. & Ho, P. C. (1985). The relationship between the human sperm hypo-osmotic swelling test, routine semen analysis and the human sperm zona-free hamster ovum penetration assay. *Fertility and Sterility*, **44**, 668–72.

Chan, S. Y. W. & Wang, C. (1987). Correlation between semen adenosine triphosphate and sperm fertilizing capacity. *Fertility and Sterility*, **47**, 717–19.

Chauhan, M., Barratt, C. L. R., Cooke, S. & Cooke, I. D. (1988). A rationalized and objective protocol for the recruitment and screening of semen donors for an AID programme. *Human Reproduction*, **3**, 773–6.

Comhaire, F. H., Vermeulen, L., Ghedira, K., Mas, J., Irvine, S. & Callipolitis, G. (1983). Adenosine triphosphate in human semen: a quantitative estimate of fertilizing potential. *Fertility and Sterility*, **40**, 500–4.

Comhaire, F. H. & Vermeulen, L. (1986). Adenosine triphosphate in semen, the zona-free hamster oocyte fusion test and male fertility. *International Journal of Andrology*, Suppl. 6, 83–7.

Cross, N. L., Morales, P., Overstreet, J. W. & Hanson, F. W. (1986). Two simple methods for detecting acrosome-reacted human sperm. *Gamete Research*, 213–26.

David, G., Czyglik, F., Mayaux, M. J. & Schwartz, D. (1980). The success of AID and semen characteristics: study on 1489 cycles and 192 ejaculates. *International Journal of Andrology*, **3**, 613–19.

David, G., Serres, C. & Jouannet, P. (1981). Kinematics of human spermatozoa. *Gamete Research*, **4**, 83–6.

De Kretser, D. M., Yates, C. & Kovacs, G. T. (1985). The use of IVF in the management of male infertility. *Clinics in Obstetrics and Gynaecology*, **12**, 767–73.

Dunphy, B. C., Kay, R., Barratt, C. L. R. & Cooke, I. D. (1989) Quality control during the conventional analysis of semen, an essential exercise. *Journal of Andrology*, **10**, 378–85.

Eliasson, R. (1971). Standards for investigation of human semen. *Andrologia*, **3**, 49–64.

Eliasson, R. (1973). Parameters of male fertility. In *Human Reproduction, Conception and Contraception*. E. S. E. Hafex and T. N. Evans, eds, pp. 39–51, Hagerstown: Harper & Row.

Eliasson, R. (1975). Analysis of semen. In *Progress of Infertility*. S. J. Behrman and R. W. Kistner, eds, pp. 691–713, Boston: Little, Brown & Co.

Eliasson, R. (1981). Analysis of semen. In *The Testis*, H. Burger and D. de Kretser, eds, pp. 381–99. New York: Raven Press.

Feneux, D., Serres, C. & Jouannet, P. (1985). Sliding spermatozoa: a dyskinesia responsible for human fertility? *Fertility and Sterility*, **44**, 508–11.

Freund, M. (1962). Inter-relationships among the characteristics of human semen and factors affecting semen specimen quality. *Journal of Reproduction and Fertility*, **4**, 143–59.

Freund, M. (1966). Standards for the rating of human sperm morphology. *International Journal of Fertility*, **4**, 143–9.

Freund, M. & Carol, B. (1964). Factors affecting haemocytometer counts of sperm concentration in human semen. *Journal of Reproduction and Fertility*, **8**, 149–55.

Freund, M. & Peterson, R. N. (1976). Semen evaluation and fertility. In *Human Semen and Fertility Regulation in Men*. E. S. E. Hafez, ed., pp. 344–54, St. Louis: C.V. Mosby Co.

Hall, J. L. (1981). Relationship between semen quality and human sperm
    penetration of zona-free hamster ova. *Fertility and Sterility*, **35**, 457–63.
Hewitt, J., Cohen, J. & Steptoe, P. (1987). Male infertility and *in-vitro*
    fertilization. In *Progress in Obstetrics and Gynaecology*. J. Studd, ed., pp.
    253–75, Edinburgh: Churchill Livingstone.
Hirsch, I., Gibbons, W. E., Lipschultz, L. T., Rassavik, K. K., Young, R. L.,
    Poindexter, A. N., Dodson, M. G. & Findley, W. E. (1986). *In-vitro*
    fertilization in couples with male factor infertility. *Fertility and Sterility*, **45**,
    659–64.
Holt, W. V., Moore, H. D. M. & Hillier, S. G. (1985). Computer assisted
    measurement of sperm swimming speed in human semen: correlation of
    results with *in-vitro* fertilization assays. *Fertility and Sterility*, **44**, 112–19.
Holt, W. V., Shenfield, F., Leonard, T., Hartman, North, R. D. & Moore, H.
    D. M. (1989). The value of sperm swimming speed measurements in
    assessing the fertility of human frozen semen. *Human Reproduction*, **4**,
    292–7.
Huszar, G. & Vigue, L. (1990) Spermatogenesis-related changes in the
    synthesis of the creatine kinase B-type and M-type isoforms in human
    spermatozoa. *Molecular Reproduction and Development*. **25**, 258–62.
Irvine, D. S. (1986). Tests of sperm function and male infertility. *Research in
    Reproduction*. **18**, 2–3.
Irvine, D. S. and Aitken, R. J. (1986). Predictive value of *in-vitro* sperm
    function tests in the context of an AID service. *Human Reproduction*, **1**,
    539–45.
Jequier, A. M. & Ukombe, E. B. (1983). Errors inherent in the performance
    of a routine semen analysis. *British Journal of Urology*, **55**, 434–6.
Jeulin, C., Feneux, D., Serres, C., Jouannet, P., Guillet-Rosso, F., Belaisch-
    Allart, J., Frydman, R. & Testart, J. (1986) Sperm factors related to
    failure of human *in-vitro* fertilization. *Journal of Reproduction and
    Fertility*, **76**, 735–44.
Jeyendran, R. S., van der Ven, H. H., Perez-Palaez, M., Crabo, B. G. &
    Zaneveld, J. D. (1984). Development of an assay to assess the functional
    integrity of the human sperm membrane and its relationship to other
    semen characteristics. *Journal of Reproduction and Fertility*, **70**, 219–28.
Katz, D. F. & Overstreet, J. W. (1980). Sperm motility assessment by
    videomicrography. *Fertility and Sterility*, **35**, 188–93.
Katz, D. F., Overstreet, J. W. & Hanson, F. W. (1980). A new quantitative
    test for sperm penetration into cervical mucus. *Fertility and Sterility*, **33**,
    179–86.
Katz, D. F., Drobnis, E. Z. & Overstreet, J. W. (1989). Factors regulating
    mammalian sperm migration through the female reproductive tract and
    oocyte vestments. *Gamete Research*, **22**, 443–69.
Kremer, J. (1965). A simple sperm penetration test. *International Journal of
    Fertility*, **10**, 209–15.
Lee, W. I., Gaddum-Rosse, P., Smith, D., Stenchever, M. & Blandau, R. J.
    (1982). Laser light-scattering study of the effect of washing on sperm
    motility. *Fertility and Sterility*, **38**, 62–7.
Lui, D. Y., du Plessis, Y. P., Nayudu, P. L., Johnston, W. I. H. & Baker, H.
    W. G. (1988). The use of *in-vitro* fertilization to evaluate putative tests of
    human sperm function. *Fertility and Sterility*, **49**, 272–7.
Mathur, S., Carlton, M., Ziegler, J., Rust, P. F. & Williamson, H. O. (1986).
    A computerised sperm motion analysis. *Fertility and Sterility*, **46**, 484–93.

Mayaux, M. J., Schwartz, D., Gzyglik, F. & David, G. (1985). Conception rate according to semen characteristics in a series of 15,364 insemination cycles: results of a multivariate analysis. *Andrologia*, **17**, 9–15.

Mayevsky, A., Dafna, B. S. & Bastoov, B. S. (1980). A multi-channel system for the measurement of spermatozoa collective motility. *International Journal of Andrology*, **3**, 436–46.

Milligan, M. P., Harris, S. & Dennis, K. J. (1980). Comparison of sperm velocity in fertile and infertile groups as measured by time-lapse photography. *Fertility and Sterility*, **34**, 509–11.

Mortimer, D., Pandya, I. J. & Sawers, R. S. (1986). Relationship between human sperm motility characteristics and sperm penetration into human cervical mucus *in-vitro*. *Journal of Reproduction and Fertility*, **78**, 93–102.

Mortimer, D., Shu, M. A. & Tan, R. (1986). Standardisation and quality control of sperm concentration and sperm motility counts in semen analysis. *Human Reproduction*, **1**, 299–303.

Mortimer, D. (1992). Objective analysis of sperm motility and kinematics. In *Handbook of Laboratory Diagnosis and Treatment of Infertility*. B. A. Keel and B. W. Webster, eds, Bocca Raton: CRC Press Inc. (In press).

Overstreet, J. W. & Katz, D. F., Hanson, F. W. & Fonseca, J. R. (1979). A simple, inexpensive method for the objective assessment of human sperm movement characteristics. *Fertility and Sterility*, **31**, 162–72.

Overstreet, J. W., Katz, D. F. (1987). Semen analysis. *Urologic Clinics of North America*, **14**, 441–9.

Pandya, I. J., Mortimer, D. & Sawers, R. S. (1986). A standardised approach for evaluating the penetration of human spermatozoa into cervical mucus *in-vitro*. *Fertility and Sterility*, **45**, 357–65.

Polansky, F.F. & Lamb, E.J. (1988). Do the results of semen analysis predict family fertility? A survival analysis study. *Fertility and Sterility*, **49**, 1059–65.

Plymate, S. R., Nagao, R. R., Muller, C. H. & Paulsen, C. A. (1987). The use of sperm penetration assay in evaluation of men with varicocele. *Fertility and Sterility*, **47**, 680–3.

Rogers, B. J. (1985). The sperm penetration assay: its usefulness re-evaluated. *Fertility and Sterility*, **43**, 821–40.

Rogers, B. J., Van Campden, H., Veno, M., Lambert, H., Bronson, R. & Hale, R. (1979). Analysis of human spermatozoa fertilizing ability using zona-free ova. *Fertility and Sterility*, **32**, 664–70.

Rogers, B. J., Perreault, S. D., Bentwood, B. J., McCarville, C., Hale, R. W. & Soderdahl, D. W. (1983). Variability in the human-hamster *in-vitro* assay for fertile evaluation. *Fertility and Sterility*, **39**, 204–11.

van Uem, J. H. M., Acosta, A. A., Swanson, R. J., Mayer, J., Ackerman, S., Burkman, I. J., Veeck, L., McDonnell, J. S., Bernadus, R. E. & Jones, H. W. Jnr. (1985). Male factor evaluation in *in-vitro* fertilization: Norfolk experience. *Fertility and Sterility*, **44**, 375–83.

Van der Ven, H. H., Jeyendran, R. S., Al-Husani, S., Perez-Pelaez, M., Diedrich, U. and Zaneveld, L. J. D. (1986). Correlation between human sperm swelling in hypo-osmotic medium (hypo-osmotic swelling test), and *in-vitro* fertilization. *Journal of Andrology*, **7**, 190–7.

World Health Organization (1980). *Laboratory Manual for the Examination of Human Semen and Semen–Cervical Mucus Interaction*. M. A. Belsey, R. Eliasson, A. J. Gallegos, K. S. Moghissi, C. A. Paulsen and M. R. N. Prasad, eds, Singapore: Press Concern.

World Health Organization (1987). WHO laboratory manual for the examination of human semen, and semen–cervical mucus interaction. Cambridge University Press.

Yanagimachi, R. (1972). Penetration of guinea pig spermatozoa into hamster eggs *in-vitro*. *Journal of Reproduction and Fertility*, **28**, 477–80.

Yanagimachi, R., Yanagimachi, H. & Rogers, B. J. (1976). The use of zona-free animal ova as a test system for the assessment of the fertilizing capacity of human spermatozoa. *Biology of Reproduction*, **15**, 471–6.

Zaini, A., Jennings, M. G. & Baker, H. W. G. (1985). Are conventional sperm morphology and motility assessments of predictive value in subfertile men? *International Journal of Andrology*, **8**, 427–35.

6

Semen cryopreservation methodology and results

B. A. KEEL and B. W. WEBSTER

Introduction

Artificial insemination with donor semen (AID) has been used successfully when clinically indicated for conditions including azoospermia, Rh
incompatibility, and genetic disorders are indicated (Beck, 1974; Karow,
1981). Bunge & Sherman (1953) first reported the use of cryopreserved
human semen for AID. Since that time, frozen human semen has been
used extensively for artificial insemination.

Cryopreserved semen has several advantages over the use of fresh
semen including ease of scheduling for both donor and patient as well as
assurance of availability of known quality donor semen. Moreover,
cryopreservation allows for the quarantining of donor semen until appropriate quality control measures can be implemented to ensure that the
ejaculate is free of infectious disease before insemination (see Greenblatt
et al., 1986). However, fewer pregnancies have been reported using
cryopreserved semen as compared to fresh semen (Steinberger & Smith,
1973; Ansbacher, 1978; Quinlivan, 1979; Smith, Rodriquez-Rigau &
Steinberger, 1981; Richter, Haning & Shapiro, 1984). Reduced fertilizing ability of cryopreserved semen has been related to ultrastructural
changes (Pederson & Lebeck, 1971), decreased penetration of cervical
mucus (Fjallbrant & Ackerman, 1969; Urry *et al.*, 1983) and decreased
post-thaw survival (Keel & Black, 1980) and motility (Smith & Steinberger, 1973; Keel & Karow, 1980; Thachil & Jewett, 1981; Keel,
Webster & Roberts, 1987; Keel & Webster, 1989).

In this chapter, the theory behind successful cryopreservation of
human semen and the methods used during this process will be reviewed.
The effects of cryopreservation on both motility characteristics and

71

function of human sperm will be examined as well as the detrimental effects of cryopreservation on the possibilities of producing a successful pregnancy.

Cryopreservation theory

The study of low temperature survival of sperm has fascinated man for more than two hundred years. The concept of banking cryopreserved human semen was first proposed in 1866 (Sherman, 1990). The emergence of the field of cryobiology has resulted in an enhanced understanding of the processes cells undergo when subjected to low temperatures and thus has led to an appreciation of the requirements of cell survival during cryopreservation. A complete discussion of these processes and requirements is beyond the scope of this chapter. The reader is referred to several reviews on this topic for further detail (Hammerstedt, Graham & Nolan, 1990; Sherman, 1990).

The major concern in successful cryopreservation of cells revolves around intracellular and extracellular water as related to (1) the formation of ice crystals and (2) the dehydration and subsequent rehydration of cells. As water is cooled below 0 °C, ice crystals begin to form. When a cell suspension (i.e. semen) is slowly cooled below 0 °C, ice crystallization occurs which initially is extracellular (Karow, 1981). The transformation of the extracellular solvent toward a more solid phase (ice formation) results in a simultaneous increase in the concentration of all other solutes in the remaining liquid phase (Hammerstedt *et al.*, 1990) thus favouring an outward osmotic diffusion of intracellular water. The vapour pressure of supercooled cellular water, which is higher than the vapour pressure of ice, creates a force that also promotes the outward movement of intracellular water (Karow, 1981). The result is cell dehydration. The rate of cooling is critical to this process and also effects both the efflux of cellular water as well as extracellular ice crystal formation. Rapid cooling favours intracellular ice crystal formation (which is usually incompatible with cell survival) and there is therefore less time for the loss of supercooled intracellular water (Karow, 1981). Thus, controlling cellular dehydration to inhibit intracellular ice crystal formation is an important step in successful cryopreservation.

With respect to human sperm cells, cryoprotectants are universally used to aid in the removal of cellular water and the protection from damage due to ice formation. Cryoprotectants can be classified in general as either penetrating (glycerol and dimethylsulphoxide, DMSO) and nonpenetrating (lactose and trehalose) based on their ability to enter cells. Both types result in cellular dehydration. They differ, however, in their ability to enter cells (Hammerstedt *et al.*, 1990). Penetrating cryoprotectants have been used extensively in the preservation of human sperm. These cryoprotectants enter the sperm and replace the intracellular water reducing the chance for intracellular ice crystal formation.

Thawing of cryopreserved cells must undergo identical but opposite processes involving a rehydration of intracellular spaces. As mentioned above, the rate of cooling is important in controlling the rate and location of ice crystal formation and degree of cell dehydration. Likewise, the rate of thawing is important for cell survival. If the cryopreserved cells are thawed too rapidly, an unbalanced rate of cryoprotectant egress and water influx occurs. On the other hand, too slow a thaw will result in recrystallization of microcrystals of intracellular water and resultant damage to cellular organelles (Hammerstedt *et al.*, 1990). In general, a greater survival of cryopreserved human sperm occurs when fairly rapid thaw rates are employed.

Cryopreservation methods

The critical areas in successful cryopreservation of human semen involve the choice of a suitable cryoprotectant and an optimized rate of freezing and thawing. Numerous reports on the use of various cryoprotectants as well as differing freezing protocols have been presented and shown to be successful. As pointed out recently in a comprehensive review by Sherman (1990), the considerable number of variables in different cryopreservation methodologies including the nature of the cryoprotectant, conditions of freezing, type of packaging, and methods for thawing, make it difficult to single out a single optimal protocol. Clearly, each laboratory must choose a protocol that is suitable and yields good results. In the next few sections, an attempt will be made to provide examples of methods that have been more successful for others.

Collection and analysis of semen

The first step in semen cryopreservation involves the collection and analysis of the ejaculate. Details of this step are provided elsewhere (Keel, 1990; see Chapter 5) and will not be discussed at length here. Briefly, semen should be collected by masturbation into a clean, dry container and delivered to the laboratory for processing within one hour after collection. Semen should be collected after 3 days of abstinence to ensure optimal quality and quantity of sperm. A complete semen analysis should next be performed to include the measurement of semen volume and sperm motility, count, morphology and, if objective analysis is possible, sperm velocity and other determinations of sperm kinematics. This 'prefreeze' data should be properly recorded for each ejaculate from each donor.

Cryoprotectants

Glycerol was the first cryoprotectant used for freezing human semen (Polge, Smith & Parkes, 1949). Glycerol continues to be the most widely used cryoprotectant in spite of the fact that a significant part of the observed reduction in sperm motility associated with cryopreservation is due to glycerol toxicity (Critser *et al.*, 1988) and that frozen-thawed sperm are osmotically damaged when removed from glycerol (Hammitt, Walker & Williamson, 1988). In fact, it has been recently reported that over 40% of commercial sperm banks today use glycerol alone (Sherman, 1990).

There is, however, an increasing use of 'extenders' in conjunction with glycerol. Most of these extenders utilize a zwitter ion buffer system composed of *N*-tris (hydroxymethyl) methyl 2-amino ethane sulphonic acid (TES) and tris (hydroxymethyl) aminomethane (TRIS), termed TEST, and contain either citrate and/or egg yolk with varying percentages of glycerol. Others contain glycerol, glycine and either sucrose or egg yolk, citrate, dextrose and glycine as cryoprotectant agents.

Several studies have examined the cryosurvival rates of human sperm preserved with various cryoprotectants. Prins and Weidel (1986) demonstrated greater progressive motility and longevity in thawed sperm when TEST–citrate–glycerol–egg yolk buffers were used. Hammitt *et al.* (1988) discovered that none of the components of egg yolk–citrate–dextrose–glycine extenders has any appreciable cryoprotective properties, while TEST–citrate buffers containing glycerol performed well. These investigators went on to report that although human semen cannot be successfully frozen in media lacking glycerol, the optimal concentration of glycerol for maintenance of maximal post-thaw fertility differs among various media and must be empirically determined (Hammitt *et al.*, 1988). In a recent study (Keel *et al.*, 1987; see below) post-thaw semen parameters were measured in ejaculates cryopreserved using 10%

glycerol compared with ejaculates preserved with TEST buffered egg yolk containing glycerol (TEST–yolk). It was concluded that the use of TEST–yolk results in ejaculates with higher post-thaw velocities, thus reducing the requirement for exceptional prefreeze velocities. Collectively, these data suggest that the use of TEST buffer containing egg yolk and glycerol may provide superior protection compared to the use of glycerol alone. In any case, it is apparent that the choice of cryoprotectant is arbitrary and that each laboratory should individually determine which provides the greatest cryosurvival.

Packaging

Once the cryoprotectant is added, the semen is either drawn into plastic paillettes (straws), or placed into glass ampules or plastic cryovials. The volume of semen in each aliquote (insemination unit) should equal approximately 0.5 to 0.8 ml. Several units may be used for a single insemination. The unit is then carefully labelled with the donor identification and date. In addition to the units which will be later thawed for insemination, a 'post-thaw unit' is also filled with a small amount of semen for determination of the post-thaw survival of the ejaculate. This post-thaw unit is usually filled last with a small amount of semen remaining after filling the other units.

The choice of the container is arbitrary. 0.5 ml straws were found to be very convenient. The units from a single ejaculate can be placed into a plastic goblet, which is also labelled with donor information. Once the semen is frozen, the goblet is placed into a cardboard screw-cap container with other ejaculates from the same donor. This container is then placed into the liquid nitrogen storage canister for long-term storage. Glass ampules and plastic cryovials are usually stored by placing them onto an aluminium cane, and the cane stored in the canister.

Freezing

The method chosen to cryopreserve semen must be one that is slow to allow effective cell dehydration and cryoprotectant influx as well as inhibit intracellular ice crystal formation. This has been accomplished by two primary methods. One involves the use of programmable mechanical freezers which precisely controls the rate of cooling (Cohen, Felten & Zeilmaker, 1981; Critser *et al.*, 1987*a*, 1988; Hammitt *et al.*, 1988). The other involves a more manual procedure utilizing refrigerated air (Keel *et* al., 1987; Keel & Webster, 1989) or liquid nitrogen vapour (Sherman, 1963; Keel & Karow, 1980; Keel & Black, 1980; Prins & Weidel, 1986; Sherman, 1990) for freezing. Both methods attempt to bring the temperature of the semen to 5 °C *slowly* followed by a more rapid reduction of temperature to that of liquid nitrogen. Numerous studies have compared these methods with varying results (Thachil & Jewett, 1981; Taylor *et al.*, 1982; Serafini & Marrs, 1986; Hammitt, Hade & Williamson, 1989). However, as pointed out recently by Sherman (1990), the basic, simple method of vapour freezing introduced nearly three decades ago (Sherman, 1963) has proved quite successful in human semen cryobanking.

Thawing

Rapid thawing to room or body temperature seems to be the optimal procedure for thawing cryopreserved human semen. This can easily be accomplished by immersing the frozen semen in room temperature or warmed water or by simply placing the semen in room air.

Summary

There are as many methods for semen cryopreservation as there are cryobanks. A general optimized method for human semen cryopreservation does not exist. Each bank should develop and optimize its own methods and procedures. As an example, the authors' own human cryopreservation program utilizes the static refrigerated air method (Keel *et al.*, 1987; Keel & Webster, 1989) which involves: (1) addition of TEST–yolk cryoprotectant, slowly in a dropwise fashion, at room temperature, (2) packaging into 0.5 ml plastic straws, (3) placing the straws horizontally at 4 °C for 30 min, followed by −85 °C (mechanical ultralow freezer) for 10 min, (4) plunging and storage into liquid nitrogen, (5) thawing by placing the straws under a stream of running luke-warm tap water.

Effects of cryopreservation on sperm function

Cryopreservation results in a marked reduction in sperm motility characteristics (Smith & Steinberger, 1973; Keel & Karow, 1980) which may be related to lower pregnancy rates reported using frozen. Several studies have presented data on the efficacy of various cryopreservation techniques for human semen (Zavos *et al.*, 1980; Thachil & Jewett, 1981; Cohen *et al.*, 1981; Taylor *et al.*, 1982; Serafini & Marrs, 1986; Prins & Weidel, 1986). However, few studies have evaluated the effects of freezing on the motility characteristics of human sperm. The commercial availability of computer assisted semen analysis systems for precise measurements of semen parameters, including velocity, has allowed reproducible and accurate description of semen characteristics (for review see Mortimer, 1990).

Microcomputerized multiple-exposure photography has been used to evaluate the effects of cryopreservation on the motility characteristics of human sperm (Keel *et al.*, 1987; Keel & Webster, 1989). Cryopreservation resulted in significant reductions in all semen parameters measured (Fig. 6.1). Sperm motility was reduced by over 50% representing a percentage recovery (survival) of 43%. Percentage recoveries of 34–76% have been reported by several previous studies (Behrman & Sawada, 1966; Smith & Steinberger, 1973; Beck & Silverstein, 1975; Keel & Black, 1980; Keel & Karow, 1980; Cohen *et al.*, 1981; Taylor *et al.*, 1982; Serafini & Marrs, 1986) and depend to a large extent upon either the cryoprotectant or the method of freezing employed.

In another study (Keel & Webster, 1989), the effects of cryopreservation were compared on semen frozen using two different cryoprotectants, glycerol and TEST–yolk. As indicated above, cryopreservation in general results in a significant reduction in all sperm parameters measured (Table 6.1). When the percentage decreases in sperm parameters as a result of cryopreservation within each group were calculated, it was obvious that sperm motility, motile density and motility index were reduced by approximately 65% regardless of the cryoprotectant employed (Table 6.2). In contrast, velocity was the least affected by cryopreservation being decreased by only 24 to 32%. Furthermore, this decrease was significantly less marked in ejaculates cryopreserved with TEST–yolk. Although these results suggest that in order to obtain post-thaw semen values suitable for artificial insemination one must use ejaculates of high prefreeze quality, the use of TEST–yolk results in ejaculates with higher post-thaw velocities. This suggests that this cryoprotectant may reduce the requirement for exceptional prefreeze semen analysis characteristics.

These studies indicate that approximately 60% of the number of motile spermatozoa will be lost as a result of cryopreservation. Although others have not demonstrated a statistical reduction in sperm

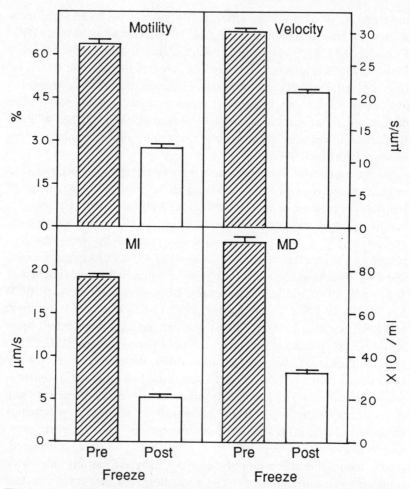

Fig. 6.1. Semen analysis data from human ejaculates before (Pre, hatched bars)
and after (Post, open bars) cryopreservation. Velocity is straight line velocity.
MI: motility index; product of the motility and the velocity. MD: motile density;
product of the motility and sperm concentration. (Data taken from Keel,
Webster & Roberts (1987). *Journal of Reproduction and Fertility*, **81**, 213.

velocity as a result of cryopreservation (Cohen *et al.*, 1981; Serafini &
Marrs, 1986), a slight decrease in velocity was observed by the authors.
However, this parameter was the least affected by the freezing process
suggesting that the average speed of sperm forward progression is the
most stable semen measure in relation to cryopreservation especially if
TEST–yolk is used as the cryoprotectant. Holt *et al.* (1989) recently
have presented data to indicate that poor maintenance of sperm velocity

Table 6.1. Semen analysis characteristics of ejaculates fresh or cryopreserved in glycerol or TEST–yolk[a]

Parameter	Fresh	Glycerol		TEST–yolk	
		Prefreeze	Post-thaw	Prefreeze	Post-thaw
Count ($\times 10^6$/ml)	89 ± 4.8^A	142 ± 3.9^B	—	90 ± 1.5^A	—
Motility (%)	$61 \pm 1.6^{C,D}$	64 ± 1.0^D	26 ± 1.1^B	59 ± 0.7^C	23 ± 0.6^A
Velocity (μm/s)	$30 \pm 0.4^{B,C}$	31 ± 0.3^C	21 ± 0.4^A	29 ± 0.2^B	22 ± 0.3^A
Motile density[b] ($\times 10^6$/ml)	55 ± 3.7^C	90 ± 3.1^D	33 ± 1.3^B	56 ± 1.3^C	22 ± 0.6^A
Motile index (μm/s)	18 ± 0.6^C	19 ± 0.4^D	5 ± 0.3^A	17 ± 0.3^B	5 ± 0.2^A
N	119	197	197	454	454

[a] Values represent mean ± standard error of the mean. Values with different superscript letters are statistically different ($P < 0.05$) by one-way analysis of variance and Duncan's test.
[b] Post-thaw motile density values increased by 10% and 100% for glycerol and TEST–yolk, respectively, to account for dilution by cryoprotectants.
Source: Data taken from Keel and Webster (1989). *Fertility and Sterility,* **52**, 100.

Table 6.2. *Cryopreservation-induced de-creases in semen analysis characteristics*

Parameter	Decrease[a]	
	Glycerol	TEST–yolk
Motility	60 ± 1.6^{C}	61 ± 1.0^{C}
Velocity	32 ± 1.6^{B}	24 ± 1.2^{A}
Motile density[b]	61 ± 1.5^{C}	57 ± 1.4^{C}
Motility index	75 ± 1.3^{D}	71 ± 1.1^{D}

[a] Percentage decrease calculated as (Pre-freeze value − Post-thaw value)/Prefreeze value × 100, mean ± standard error of the mean. Values with different superscript letters are statistically different ($P < 0.01$) by one-way analysis of variance and Duncan's test.

[b] Post-thaw motile densities values increased by 10% and 100% for glycerol and TEST–yolk, respectively, to account for dilution by cryoprotectants.

Source: Data taken from Keel and Webster (1989). *Fertility and Sterility*, **52**, 100.

following cryopreservation was associated with a significant decrease in fecundity pointing to the importance of preserving this parameter in cryopreserved sperm.

Significant variation in semen parameters within individuals has been reported (Poland *et al.*, 1985). Likewise, significant differences have also been noted in the sensitivity of semen from different donors to the effects of cryopreservation. In general, most donors display a similar percentage decrease in motility, velocity, motility index and motile density as a result of freezing, but, as shown in Table 6.3, there can be notable exceptions. For example, Donor A exhibited a greater resistance to changes in motility, motility index, and motile density, while semen from Donor B proved to be the most sensitive to cryopreservation. These data indicate that considerable variation exists in the ability of sperm from individual donors to survive the rigours of cryopreservation and point to the difficulty in predicting the outcome of ejaculates subjected to freeze–thaw procedures.

Virtually all ejaculates evaluated have prefreeze sperm parameters which were in the 'normal range'. Cryopreservation not only resulted in a significant reduction in these parameters but also markedly shifted the

Table 6.3. *Percentage change* of semen data amongst five donors after cryopreservation of the semen*

Donor	Motility	Velocity	Motility index	Motile density
A ($n = 24$)	32.5 ± 5^{bc}	31 ± 3^{bc}	51 ± 6^d	41 ± 3^C
B ($n = 20$)	70 ± 2^e	35 ± 2^{bc}	82 ± 1^f	73 ± 2^{ef}
C ($n = 55$)	52 ± 2^d	30 ± 2^b	69 ± 2^e	57 ± 2^d
D ($n = 10$)	55 ± 5^d	0.2 ± 9^a	61 ± 5^{de}	61 ± 6^{de}
E ($n = 14$)	54 ± 9^d	33 ± 3^{bc}	76 ± 3^{ef}	72 ± 3^{ef}
All ($n = 164$)	57 ± 2	30 ± 2	72 ± 2	62 ± 2

* (Prefreeze value − post-thaw value)/prefreeze value × 100.
   Values are expressed as the mean ± s.e. Means identified by different superscript letters are statistically different ($P < 0.05$) by one-way ANOVA and Duncan's test.
Source: Data taken from Keel, Webster and Roberts (1987). *Journal of Reproduction and Fertility*, **81**, 213.

values into the 'subnormal' or 'suboptimal' range (Fig. 6.2). Suboptimal semen parameters are most often cited as the reason for the reported reduced fertility potential of cryopreserved semen.

Numerous reports have examined the fertilizing ability of frozen-thawed semen using the zona-free hamster egg penetration assay. Conflicting results exist with some investigators reporting lower penetration rates with frozen sperm (Binor, Sokoloski & Wolf, 1980; Laufer *et al.*, 1984) while others report comparable penetration rates between fresh and frozen sperm (Urry *et al.*, 1983; Serafini & Marrs, 1986). Still others have shown variable results depending upon the cryoprotectant used and the freezing protocols employed (Cohen *et al.*, 1981; Jeyendran *et al.*, 1984; Critser *et al.*, 1987a,b; Hammitt *et al.*, 1988). Much of the controversy centers around the interpretation of the sperm penetration assay. Laufer *et al.* (1984) demonstrated that despite a greater than 50% reduction in penetration rates as a result of cryopreservation, 75% of the frozen–thawed samples maintained a penetration rate exceeding 14%, the lower limit of 'normal' fertilizing capacity in that laboratory. Urry *et al.* (1983) also showed that if a lower limit of 20–25% penetration is used, only 6% of sperm samples in their study declined from a penetration rate considered normal to a subfertile value following freezing. Furthermore, if 10% is used as the cut off (which has been proposed in some studies), none of the samples decreased from the normal to subfertile range (Urry *et al.*, 1983).

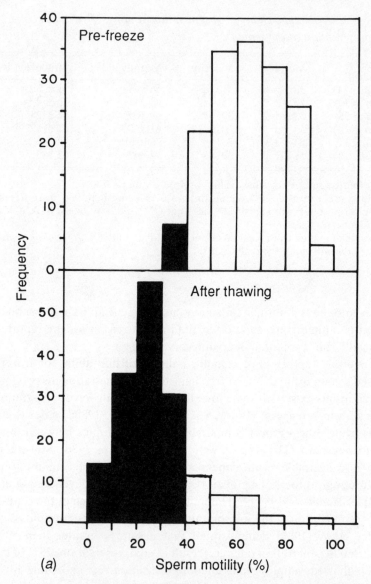

Fig. 6.2. Frequency distribution histogram displaying the number of ejaculates (frequency) having prefreeze (top) and post-thaw (bottom) values for (*a*) sperm motility; (*b*) sperm velocity; (*c*) motility index; and (*d*) motile density. Open bars refer to ejaculates having normal values; close bars refer to ejaculates having subnormal values. (Data taken from Keel, Webster & Roberts (1987). *Journal of Reproduction and Fertility*, **81**, 213 with permission.)

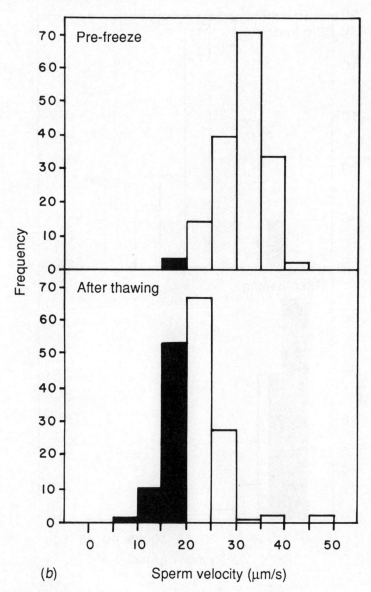

(b)   Sperm velocity (μm/s)

Fig. 6.2 (b).

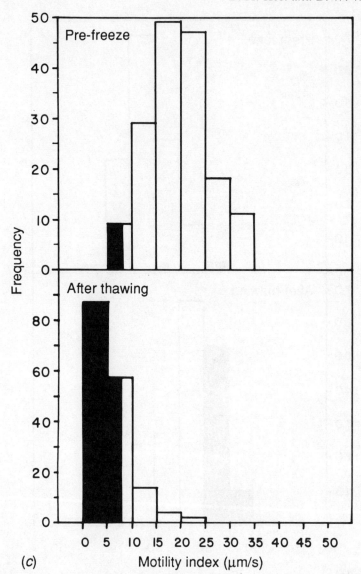

Fig. 6.2 (c).

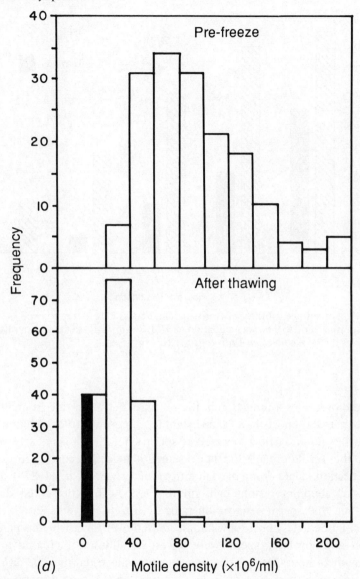

(d)

Fig. 6.2 (d).

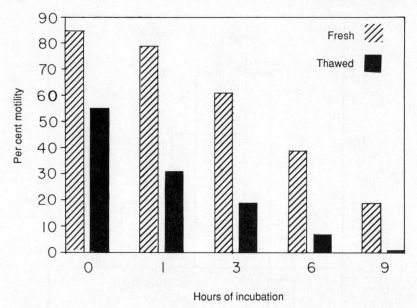

Fig. 6.3. Percentage motility of fresh (hatched bars) and frozen-thawed (solid bars) sperm after 0 to 9 hours incubation at 37 °C *in vitro*. (Data taken from Keel & Black (1980). *Archives in Andrology*, **4**, 213.

Therefore, does a reduction in the sperm penetration rate from 80% prefreeze to 25% post-thaw (as an example) represent a true reduction in the fertility potential of cryopreserved sperm since the 30% is clearly well above the 'fertile range'? Further research is indeed needed to answer this question. Data from the laboratory of Critser *et al.* (1987*b*) do, however, shed interesting light on this issue. They presented data indicating that sperm penetration rates by frozen–thawed sperm were highest immediately post-thaw and decreased over time, whereas penetration rates by fresh sperm were lowest initially and increased to a maximum 24 hours later. These investigators suggested that the differences in penetration rates over time between cryopreserved sperm and their fresh counterparts may be due to differences in their initial acrosomal status and the time requirements for capacitation.

Other investigators have universally demonstrated a significant decrease in the ability of cryopreserved sperm to penetrate bovine cervical mucus (Zavos & Cohen, 1980; Urry *et al.*, 1983; Gehring, 1987), human cervical mucus (Fjallbrant & Ackerman, 1969), and 'synthetic mucus' (polyacrylamide gel, Goldstein *et al.*, 1982) *in vitro*. This decrease may be related to an observed reduction in the motility longevity of cryopreserved sperm (Fig. 6.3) suggesting that cryopreservation may affect the ability of thawed sperm to maintain motility *in vivo*. Taken together these data suggest that the physiology of cryopreserved sperm is sufficiently different from fresh sperm to cause a narrowing of the 'window' of fertilizability of frozen sperm, as has been suggested by Critser *et al.* (1987*b*). It can thus be concluded from these data that the timing of the insemination using frozen–thawed sperm is critical to ensure that the sperm is deposited as closely as possible to the time of ovulation.

Fecundity of cryopreserved sperm

Numerous studies have reported on the efficacy and fecundity of fresh (Steinberger & Smith, 1973; Chong & Taymor, 1975; Dixon & Buttram, 1976; Ansbacher, 1978; Sulewski, Eisenberg & Stenger, 1978; Quinlivan, 1979; Glezerman, 1981; Smith *et al.*, 1981; Aiman, 1982; Albrecht, Cramer & Schiff, 1982; Corson, 1980; Richter *et al.*, 1984; Bordson *et al.*, 1986; Meeks *et al.*, 1986) and frozen (Steinberger & Smith, 1973; Ansbacher, 1978; Sulewski *et al.*, 1978; Quinlivan, 1979; David *et al.*, 1980; Smith *et al.*, 1981; Trounson *et al.*, 1981; Emperaire, Gauzere-Somireu & Audebert, 1982; Richter *et al.*, 1984; Thorneycroft, Bustillo & Marik, 1984; Bordson *et al.*, 1986) AID. The results of these studies are summarized in Table 6.4. Clearly, caution must be exercised when pooling the results of these studies since different insemination protocols were employed and varying numbers of patients and AI cycles were evaluated. In general, though, it can be concluded that fresh AID results in a 20–30% greater raw and cumulative pregnancy rate and 5% greater monthly fecundity rate compared with frozen AID.

Several studies have suggested that the reported decreased fecundity of frozen semen may be related to a cryopreservation-induced reduction in sperm motility and survival as indicated above. This has led several investigators to compare data from successful and unsuccessful AI cycles (David *et al.*, 1980; Aiman, 1982; Keel & Webster, 1989) to determine if and/or what semen characteristics were a factor in the success of AID. This possibility has been examined by comparing semen data from ejaculates resulting in conception, either fresh or frozen using glycerol or TEST–yolk (Keel & Webster, 1989). The post-thaw data were statistically identical in cycle of conception (COC) ejaculates regardless of the

Table 6.4. *Summation of published studies on raw, cumulative and monthly fecundity of fresh and frozen AID*

Author	Fresh AID			Frozen AID		
	Raw %	Cum. preg. rate %	Monthly fecundity %	Raw %	Cum. preg. rate %	Monthly fecundity %
Meeks et al., 1986	58	97[d]	15[a]			
Albrecht et al., 1982	64[c]	85[d]	15[a]			
Aiman, 1982	80	80[c,e]	14[a,c]			
Glezerman, 1981	85	97[d]	15[a,c]			
Corson, 1980	75	80[d]	12[a,c]			
Dixon & Buttram, 1976	45	—	13[b,c]			
Chong & Taymor, 1975	72	90[c,d]	16[a,c]			
Trounson et al., 1981				47[c]	64[d]	9[a,c]
David et al., 1980				37[c]	—	11[b]
Thorneycroft et al., 1984				42[c]	—	12[a]
Emperaine et al., 1982				64	—	9[b]
Steinberger & Smith, 1973	73	—	11[b,c]	61	—	9[b,c]
Smith et al., 1981	74	73[e]	20[a,c]	60	60[e]	8[a,c]
Richter et al., 1984	40[c]	93[d]	19[b]	18[c]	45[d]	5[b]
Bordson et al., 1986	16[c]	—	12[b]	14[c]	—	10[b]
Keel & Webster, 1989	19	54[d]	12[b]	18	37[d]	6[b]
Mean ± SEM	58 ± 7	83 ± 4	14 ± 1	40 ± 7	52 ± 6	9 ± 1

[a] Monthly fecundity calculated as the average of each month's pregnancy rate.
[b] Monthly fecundity calculated as the total number of pregnancies divided by the total number of AI cycles.
[c] Value calculated from the data presented by the respective authors.
[d] 12 month cumulative pregnancy rate.
[e] 10 month cumulative pregnancy rate.

cryoprotectant used (Table 6.5). In marked contrast, the COC post-thaw motility, velocity, and motility index were significantly reduced by 1.4- to 3-fold compared with the fresh COC ejaculates.

In comparing the fresh and post-thaw data from successful AI cycles, the total number of motile sperm inseminated in the cryopreserved group was 5- to 6-fold lower than the patients receiving fresh semen. A reduction in the number of motile sperm could explain the decreased fecundity of frozen sperm reported by others. Richter *et al.* (1984), in an elegantly designed study in which the patients received fresh or frozen semen in alternating cycles (thus the patient served as her own control), observed that the fertility potential of fresh semen was three times greater than the frozen counterpart. However, these authors recognized that their minimum post-thaw semen analysis criteria (at least 9×10^6 motile sperm/AI) may not have been adequate and may have led to their low success rate. These investigators later presented data indicating a significant increase in pregnancy rates when greater than 100 million motile sperm are inseminated than when less than that number are inseminated in the first cycle when frozen semen is used (Brown, Boone & Shapiro, 1988). In support of this, Bordson *et al.* (1986) observed no differences in the fecundity of fresh and frozen semen when at least 40×10^6 motile sperm were inseminated. Therefore, the fecundity of frozen semen may be dependent on the number of motile semen inseminated.

No differences have been observed, however, in the fecundity of frozen AI compared with fresh AI. Furthermore, no differences have been observed in fecundity of cryopreserved semen regardless of the cryoprotectant employed (Table 6.6). It was observed that pregnancy rates using TEST–yolk–preserved semen were not statistically different from either the fresh or glycerol groups. These results indicate that TEST–yolk–preserved semen is at least as effective as glycerol-preserved semen in producing pregnancies. Indeed, the pregnancy rates were very similar to fresh semen. The fact that the use of TEST–yolk allows for the acceptance of ejaculates with prefreeze semen values significantly reduced compared with the glycerol group (see Table 6.1), and that the use of TEST–yolk results in improved post-thaw velocities (see Table 6.2) and adequate pregnancy rates indicates that this cryoprotectant may offer advantages over the use of glycerol alone.

Statistically similar fecundities in the fresh and frozen group were observed in the face of markedly increased number of motile sperm in the fresh group. Clearly, these results should not be interpreted to

Table 6.5. *Semen analysis data from fresh and TEST–yolk and glycerol frozen semen resulting in pregnancy*[a]

Parameter	Fresh	Glycerol		TEST–yolk	
		Prefreeze	Post-thaw	Prefreeze	Post-thaw
Count ($\times 10^6$/ml)	92 ± 14.1[a]	152 ± 15.6[B]	—	103 ± 5.1[A]	—
Motility (%)	65 ± 3.9[b]	66 ± 3.4[B]	35 ± 4.1[B]	62 ± 2.4[B]	28 ± 2.2[A]
Velocity (μm/s)	33 ± 0.9[C]	32 ± 0.7[C]	23 ± 1.8[A]	27 ± 1.1[B]	23 ± 0.8[A]
Motile density[b] ($\times 10^6$/ml)	58 ± 9.2[b,C]	101 ± 13.6[D]	42 ± 3.1[A,B]	62 ± 3.8[C]	36 ± 2.6[A]
Motile index (μm/s)	21 ± 1.5[C]	20 ± 1.3[C]	8 ± 1.4[A]	16 ± 1.1[B]	6 ± 0.6[A]
Artificial insemination motile density (10^6/AI)	132 ± 24.4[B]	—	24 ± 1.7[A]	—	25 ± 0.8[A]
N	14	18	18	29	30

[a] Mean $\pm$ SEM. Values with different superscript letters are statistically different ($P < 0.05$) by one-way ANOVA and Duncan's test.

[b] Post-thaw MD values increased by 10% and 100% for glycerol and TEST–yolk, respectively, to account for dilution by cryoprotectants.

Source: Data taken from Keel and Webster (1989). *Fertility and Sterility,* **52,** 100.

Table 6.6. *Pregnancy rates of patients inseminated with fresh and cryopreserved semen*

	Fresh	Glycerol	TEST–yolk	Glycerol and TEST–yolk combined
Total number of patients/group	67	97	112	209
Number insemination cycles	310	405	512	917
Average cycles/patient	4.63	4.17	4.57	4.38
Number patients pregnant	18	17	27	44
Monthly fecundity rate[a]	5.8%	4.2%	5.3%	4.8%
Raw pregnancy rate[b]	26.9%	17.5%	24.1%	21.0%
Cumulative pregnancy rate[c]	52.9%	27.1%	68.5%	62.4%

[a] Number of pregnancies/number of AID cycles.
[b] Number of pregnancies/number of patients.
[c] Cumulative over 14 cycles. Not significantly different by Mantel-Byar life-table analysis.
Source: Data taken from Keel and Webster (1989). *Fertility and Sterility,* **52**, 100.

indicate that the overall quality of the ejaculate, both fresh and frozen, is not important in determining the outcome of AID. These results do, however, suggest that frozen ejaculates having an artificial insemination motile density (i.e. the total number of motile sperm inseminated) of at least 20×10^6 give statistically similar success rates as fresh ejaculates containing on average five times the number of motile sperm inseminated. It is conceivable that 20 million motile sperm may be the minimum number of motile sperm needed for successful AID. Whether increasing this 40×10^6/AI as defined by Bordson *et al.* (1986) will increase the fecundity of frozen semen remains to be determined.

Conclusion

Many factors can influence the success of an AID program including the physical condition of the recipient, methods used for AI timing, number of inseminations/cycle, drop out rate, and choice and quality of ejaculate. Cryopreservation of donor semen allows for quarantining and quality assessment of the ejaculate before the patient is exposed to the ejaculate. The very real danger of infecting a recipient with HIV and other devastating, although less lethal, diseases speaks clearly to the need for offering only frozen AID to patients. There is an urgent need for more data on the effectiveness of cryopreserved semen for AID and on the minimum number of motile sperm required per insemination. However, the results of numerous investigations indicate that although the overall quality of cryopreserved sperm may be reduced, if a minimum criteria for ejaculate quality is established and accurate methods are employed to determine insemination timing, the use of cryopreserved semen can offer a viable, effective, and relatively safe alternative to AID with fresh semen.

Acknowledgements

The authors would like to thank the following team members who have provided outstanding technical and clinical assistance: Kris Zumbach, Nancy Jabara, Toni Clinton, Michelle McShane, Vicki Roberts, Cathy Robertson, Cindy Stewart and Joleen Zivnuska. Their dedication toward quality work is greatly appreciated. Work in the authors' laboratory was supported in part by the Women's Research Institute,

HCA/Wesley Medical Center and the Wesley Foundation, Wichita, Kansas.

References

Aiman, J. (1982). Factors affecting the success of donor insemination. *Fertility and Sterility*, **37**, 94–9.
Albrecht, B. H., Cramer, D. & Schiff, I. (1982). Factors influencing the success of artificial insemination. *Fertility and Sterility*, **37**, 792–7.
Ansbacher, R. (1978). Artificial insemination with frozen spermatozoa. *Fertility and Sterility*, **29**, 375–9.
Beck, W. W. (1974). Artificial insemination and semen preservation. *Clinical Obstetrics and Gynecology*, **17**, 115–25.
Beck, W. W. & Silverstein, I. (1975). Variable motility recovery of spermatozoa following freeze preservation. *Fertility and Sterility*, **26**, 863–7.
Behrman, S. J. & Sawada, Y. (1966). Heterologous and homologous inseminations with human semen frozen and stored in a liquid nitrogen refrigerator. *Fertility and Sterility*, **17**, 457–66.
Binor, Z., Sokoloski, J. E. & Wolf, D. P. (1980). Penetration of the zona-free hamster egg by human sperm. *Fertility and Sterility*, **33**, 321–7.
Bordson, B. L., Ricci, E., Dickey, R. P., Dunaway, H., Taylor, S. N. & Curole, D. N. (1986). Comparison of fecundability with fresh and frozen semen in therapeutic donor insemination. *Fertility and Sterility*, **46**, 466–9.
Brown, C. A., Boone, W. R. & Shapiro, S. S. (1988). Improved cryopreserved semen fecundability in an alternating fresh-frozen artificial insemination program. *Fertility and Sterility*, **50**, 325–7.
Bunge, R. G. & Sherman, J. K. (1953). Fertilizing capacity of frozen human spermatozoa. *Nature*, London, **172**, 767–8.
Chong, A. P. & Taymor, M. L. (1975). Sixteen years experience with therapeutic donor insemination. *Fertility and Sterility*, **26**, 791–5.
Cohen, J., Felten, P. & Zeilmaker, G. H. (1981). *In vitro* fertilizing capacity of fresh and cryopreserved human spermatozoa: a comparative study of freezing and thawing procedures. *Fertility and Sterility*, **36**, 356–62.
Corson, S. L. (1980). Factors affecting donor artifical insemination success rates. *Fertility and Sterility*, **33**, 415–22.
Critser, J. K., Huse-Benda, A. R., Aaker, D. V., Arneson, B. W. & Ball, G. D. (1987*a*). Cryopreservation of human spermatozoa. I. Effects of holding procedure and seeding on motility, fertilizability, and acrosome reaction. *Fertility and Sterility*, **47**, 656–63.
Critser, J. K., Arneson, B. W., Aaker, D. V., Huse-Benda, A. R. & Ball, G. D. (1987*b*). Cryopreservation of human spermatozoa. II. Post-thaw chronology of motility and of zona-free hamster ova penetration. *Fertility and Sterility*, **47**, 980–4.
Critser, J. D., Huse-Benda, A. R., Aaker, D. V., Arneson, B. W. & Ball, G. D. (1988). Cryopreservation of human spermatozoa. III. The effect of cryoprotectants on motility. *Fertility and Sterility*, **50**, 314–20.
David, G., Czyglik, F., Mayaux, M. J. & Schwartz, D. (1980). The success of AID and semen characteristics: study on 1489 cycles and 192 ejaculates. *International Journal of Andrology*, **3**, 613–19.

Dixon, R. E. & Buttram, V. C. (1976). Artificial insemination using donor semen: a review of 171 cases. *Fertility and Sterility*, **27**, 130–4.

Emperaire, J. C., Gauzere-Soumireu, E. & Audebert, A. J. M. (1982). Female fertility and donor insemination. *Fertility and Sterility*, **37**, 90–3.

Fjallbrant, B. & Ackerman, D. R. (1969). Cervical mucus penetration *in vitro* by fresh and frozen-preserved human semen specimens. *Journal of Reproduction and Fertility*, **20**, 515–17.

Gehring, W. G. (1987). Bovine mucus penetration test and routine semen analysis of fresh and cryopreserved human spermatozoa. *Andrologia*, **19**, 544–50.

Glezerman, M. (1981). Two hundred and seventy cases of artificial donor insemination: management and results. *Fertility and Sterility*, **35**, 180–7.

Goldstein, M. C., Wix, L. S., Foote, R. H., Feldschuh, R. & Feldschuh, J. (1982). Migration of fresh and cryopreserved human spermatozoa in polyacrylamide gel. *Fertility and Sterility*, **37**, 668–74.

Greenblatt, R. M., Handsfield, H. H., Sayers, M. H. & Holmes, K. K. (1986). Screening therapeutic insemination donors for sexually transmitted diseases; overview and recommendations. *Fertility and Sterility*, **46**, 356–64.

Hammerstedt, R. H., Graham, J. K. & Nolan, J. P. (1990). Cryopreservation of mammalian sperm: what we ask them to survive. *Journal of Andrology*, **11**, 73–88.

Hammitt, D. G., Walker, D. L. & Williamson, R. A. (1988). Concentration of glycerol required for optimal survival and *in vitro* fertilizing capacity of frozen sperm is dependent on cryopreservation medium. *Fertility and Sterility*, **49**, 680–7.

Hammitt, D. G., Hade, D. K. & Williamson, R. A. (1989). Survival of human sperm following controlled- and noncontrolled-rate cryopreservation. *Andrologia*, **21**, 311–17.

Holt, W. V., Shenfield, F., Leonard, T., Hartman, T. D., North, R. D. & Moore, H. D. M. (1989). The value of sperm swimming speed measurements in assessing the fertility of human frozen semen. *Human Reproduction*, **4**, 292–7.

Jeyendran, R. S., Van Der Ven, H. H., Kennedy, W., Perez-Pelaez, M. & Zaneveld, L. J. D. (1984). Comparison of glycerol and a zwitter ion buffer system as cryoprotective media for human spermatozoa. *Journal of Andrology*, **5**, 1–7.

Karow, A.M., Jr. (1981). Human gametes. In *Organ Preservation for Transplantation*, 2nd edn., A. M. Karow, Jr. & D. E. Pegg, eds., Marcel Dekker, New York.

Keel, B. A. & Black, J. B. (1980). Reduced motility longevity in thawed human spermatozoa. *Archives of Andrology*, **4**, 213–15.

Keel, B. A. & Karow, A. M. (1980). Motility characteristics of human sperm, nonfrozen and cryopreserved. *Archives of Andrology*, **4**, 205–12.

Keel, B. A. (1990). The semen analysis. In *Handbook of the Laboratory Diagnosis and Treatment of Infertility*, B. A. Keel and B. W. Webster, eds, pp. 27–69, Boca Raton: CRC Press, Inc.

Keel, B. A. & Webster, B. W. (1989). Semen analysis data from fresh and cryopreserved donor ejaculates: comparison of cryoprotectants and pregnancy rates. *Fertility and Sterility*, **52**, 100–5.

Keel, B. A., Webster, B. W. & Roberts, D. K. (1987). Effects of cryopreservation on the motility characteristics of human spermatozoa. *Journal of Reproduction and Fertility*, **81**, 213–20.

Laufer, N., Margalioth, E. J., Navot, D., Shemesh, A. & Schenker, J. G. (1984). Reduced penetration of zona-free hamster ova by cryopreserved human spermatozoa. *Archives of Andrology*, **14**, 217–22.

Meeks, G. R., McDonald, J., Gookin, K. & Bates, G. W. (1986). Insemination with fresh donor semen. *Obstetrics and Gynecology*, **68**, 527–30.

Mortimer, D. (1990). Objective analysis of sperm motility and kinematics. In *Handbook of the Laboratory Diagnosis and Treatment of Infertility*, B.A. Keel & B. W. Webster, eds, pp. 97–134, Boca Raton: CRC press, Inc.

Pederson, H. & Lebeck, P. E. (1971). Ultrastructural changes in the human spermatozoa after freezing for artificial insemination. *Fertility and Sterility*, **22**, 125–33.

Poland, M. L., Moghissi, K. S., Giblin, P. T., Ager, J. W. & Olson, J. M. (1985). Variation of semen measures within normal men. *Fertility and Sterility*, **44**, 396–400.

Polge, C., Smith, A. U. & Parkes, A. S. (1949). Revival of spermatozoa after vitrification and dehydration at low temperatures. *Nature*, London, **164**, 666.

Prins, G. S. & Weidel, L. (1986). A comparative study of buffer systems as cryoprotectants for human spermatozoa. *Fertility and Sterility*, **46**, 147–9.

Quinlivan, W. L. (1979). Therapeutic donor insemination: results and causes of nonfertilization. *Fertility and Sterility*, **32**, 157–60.

Richter, M. A., Haning, R. V. & Shapiro, S. S. (1984). Artificial donor insemination: fresh versus frozen semen; the patient as her own control. *Fertility and Sterility*, **41**, 277–80.

Serafini, P. & Marrs, R. P. (1986). Computerized staged-freezing technique improves sperm survival and preserves penetration of zona-free hamster ova. *Fertility and Sterility* **45**, 854–8.

Sherman, J. K. (1963). Improved methods of preservation of human spermatozoa by freezing and freeze-drying. *Fertility and Sterility*, **14**, 49–54.

Sherman, J. K. (1990). Cryopreservation of human semen. In *Handbook of the Laboratory Diagnosis and Treatment of Infertility*, B. A. Keel & B. W. Webster, eds, pp. 229–60, Boca Raton: CRC Press, Inc.

Smith, K. D. & Steinberger, E. (1973). Survival of spermatozoa in a human sperm bank. *Journal of the American Medical Association*, **223**, 774–7.

Smith, K. D., Rodriquez-Rigau, L. J. & Steinberger, E. (1981). The influence of ovulatory dysfunction and timing of insemination on the success of artificial insemination donor (AID) with fresh or cryopreserved semen. *Fertility and Sterility*, **36**, 496–502.

Steinberger, E. & Smith, K. D. (1973). Artificial insemination with fresh or frozen semen. *Journal of the American Medical Association*, **223**, 778–83.

Sulewski, J. M., Eisenberg, F. & Stenger, V. G. (1978). A longitudinal analysis of artificial insemination with donor semen. *Fertility and Sterility*, **29**, 527–31.

Taylor, P. J., Wilson, J., Laycock, R. & Webster, J. (1982). A comparison of freezing and thawing methods for the cryopreservation of human semen. *Fertility and Sterility*, **37**, 100–3.

Thachil, J. V. & Jewett, M. A. (1981). Preservation techniques for human semen. *Fertility and Sterility*, **35**, 546–8.

Thorneycroft, I. H., Bustillo, M. & Marik, J. (1984). Donor fertility in an artificial insemination program. *Fertility and Sterility*, **41**, 144–5.

Trounson, A. O., Matthews, C. D. & Kovacs, G. T. (1981). Artificial insemination by frozen donor semen: results of multicentre Australian experience. *International Journal of Andrology*, **4**, 227–34.

Urry, R. L., Carrell, D. T., Hull, D. B., Middleton, R. G. & Wiltbank, M. D. (1983). Penetration of zona-free hamster ova and bovine cervical mucus by fresh and frozen human spermatozoa. *Fertility and Sterility*, **39**, 690–4.

Zavos, P. M., Goodpasture, J. C., Zaneveld, L. J. & Cohen, M. R. (1980). Motility and enzyme activity of human spermatozoa stored for 24 hours at +5 degrees Celsius and −196 degrees Celsius. *Fertility and Sterility*, **34**, 607–9.

Zavos, P. M. & Cohen, M. R. (1980). Bovine mucus penetration test: an assay for fresh and cryopreserved human spermatozoa. *Fertility and Sterility*, **34**, 175–6.

7

Ovulation timing

E. A. LENTON

Introduction

Donor insemination (DI) along with many of the new assisted reproductive technologies requires an accurate knowledge of the time of
follicle rupture or ovulation in order to optimize its effectiveness in the
treatment of infertility. Recent advances in assay techniques, particularly
the development of monoclonal antibody-based immunoradiometric or
enzyme-linked immunosorbent assay systems which confer precision,
simplicity and speed on the measurement of hormone concentrations in
either plasma or urine have now made this a practical possibility.

The human reproductive cycle

The reproductive cycle in the human female is well characterized. During
the first week, one or occasionally two follicles are selected from a larger
cohort of recruited follicles and under the influence of trophic stimulation
(follicle stimulating hormone, FSH and luteinizing hormone, LH) from
the pituitary, develop to become the dominant follicle/s destined to
ovulate at mid-cycle (approximately Day 14). As the dominant follicle
develops, it secretes increasing quantities of oestradiol into the periph-
eral circulation in proportion to its increasing size (volume).

The mature pre-ovulatory follicle is able to initiate a rapid increase in
LH concentrations, known as the LH surge which brings about a number
of changes within the follicle thus preparing it for ovulation (Fig. 7.1).
One of these changes is a shift in the synthetic potential of the granulosa
cells lining the follicle from oestradiol to progesterone secretion, so
concentrations of oestradiol within the still-intact follicle fall, whilst those
of progesterone rise. Also in response to the rapidly rising LH concentrations, the oocyte resumes meiosis in anticipation of fertilization, and

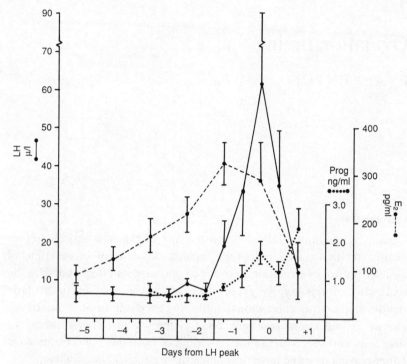

Fig. 7.1. Geometric means and 68% confidence intervals of LH, oestradiol and progesterone during the late follicular phase and over the spontaneous LH surge in 6 normally ovulating women. Blood samples were obtained twice daily, at 0800 and 2000 h.

the basement membrane of the follicle undergoes degenerative changes in preparation for rupture (ovulation). In parallel with the changing intra-follicular oestradiol : progesterone concentrations are similar changes in circulating steroid levels which can, of course, be monitored by plasma or urine sampling. Following ovulation, the follicular remnants survive as corpora lutea producing steroid hormones which support the second half of the cycle thus ensuring optimum conditions for implantation and pregnancy should the oocyte have been successfully fertilized.

To summarize those changes in the reproductive cycle which are relevant for ovulation timing: during the period that the follicle is developing, and up to the onset of the LH surge, the cells associated with the follicle (both theca outside the follicle and granulosa cells contained within the basement membrane) secrete increasing amounts of oestradiol which in turn initiate changes in the cervix and in the cervical mucus.

These changes, which can be quantified as alterations in the volume and spinnbarkeit of the mucus, have the function of optimizing the passage of spermatozoa through the reproductive tract at a time when there is the greatest probability of encountering an egg.

With the onset of the LH surge, oestradiol secretion declines and progesterone increases as shown in Fig. 7.1, indirectly giving rise to the familiar mid-cycle increase in basal body temperature. However, it is also known that progesterone reverses the mucus changes brought about by oestradiol such that the cervix rapidly becomes impenetrable to spermatozoa; so rising progesterone levels signal the end of the fertile phase. Thus there are a number of easily defined hormonal changes (oestradiol, progesterone, LH – Templeton, Penney & Lees, 1982) or indirect indices of these hormone changes (follicle volume, cervical mucus, BBT – Leader, Wiseman & Taylor, 1985) whose changes during the pre-ovulatory period could, theoretically, be used to time insemination.

Prediction of ovulation

It is clear that the events described in Fig. 7.1 could be considered to represent an 'ovulation window' whereby, as the follicle matures, changes in the reproductive tract permit sperm to penetrate through the cervix.

This represents an opening of the 'window', and the sperm that gained access may well survive within the tubal environment for some considerable time waiting for ovulation and the release of the oocyte. Release of the egg is co-ordinated by the LH surge and occurs at a fairly precise interval following the onset of this signal. The LH surge also signals the oestradiol : progesterone shift and thus indirectly determines the end of the 'ovulation window'. The duration of the ovulation window may be as long as 5 days, or as short as 12 hours, and will vary from individual to individual. In some women, several days each cycle are characterized by good quality mucus whilst in others the duration of pre-ovulatory type mucus may be only a few hours. While both extremes pose problems for donor insemination clinics, they would not necessarily impede spontaneous or unassisted conception because normal spermatozoa can survive for several days under favourable conditions. Unfortunately, cryopreserved sperm do not have the longevity of fresh sperm (Smith, Rodriquez-Rigau & Steinberger, 1981; Richter, Haning & Shapiro, 1984) and must be inseminated within a few hours of ovulation. Thus for present-day donor insemination clinics, where only cryopreserved sperm is permissible, it becomes imperative to determine not only when the ovulation window is open but also to predict in advance when it will close, so that insemination is performed as close to, but always before, the event of ovulation as is practicable.

In the past, methods of hormone monitoring have always been considered expensive (requiring endocrine laboratories, trained technicians) as well as being slow, complex to interpret and disruptive from the patient's point of view. Many donor insemination clinics have instead utilized the cheaper but more indirect methods of timing inseminations, possibly without fully appreciating the drawbacks associated with them particularly when cryopreserved sperm are utilized.

Indirect predictors of ovulation

Basal body temperature

One of the earliest methods used to monitor ovulation for donor insemination was basal body temperature recording (BBT). Unfortunately this extremely simple and inexpensive technique is difficult to perform accurately (Quagliarello & Arny, 1986) and requires considerable compliance by the patient (Partenteau-Carreau, 1981). Furthermore, although changes in a basal body temperature record can denote an ovulatory cycle (Lenton, Weston & Cooke, 1977), they cannot be used to predict ovulation because the direct signal responsible for the rise in temperature (the increase in progesterone) occurs very late in the 'ovulation window' and is, in fact, the event that closes the window. Thus, by the time a rise in basal body temperature has been observed and reported to the clinic, the optimum time for insemination has passed.

Cervical mucus assessment

For many years, assessment of the changes in cervical mucus (Insler, Melamed & Eichenbrenner, 1972) was universally accepted as the easiest method to time inseminations (Kovacs *et al.*, 1988). A significant advantage is that mucus assessment does not require any sample collection by the patient or trained personnel other than the inseminating nurse or clinician. However, the technique does require patients to attend the clinic frequently during the mid-cycle period for repeated vaginal examinations while interpretation of the mucus changes is somewhat subjective. There are, however, serious limitations to the universal efficacy of cervical mucus assessments due, for the most part, to the indirect nature of the connection between mucus changes and ovulation. As explained above, mucus changes are brought about by rising concentrations of oestradiol associated with the development of the dominant follicle and are not directly related to its ultimate rupture. The magnitude and duration of the cervical mucus changes will vary from individual to individual just as the amount of oestradiol, the size of the follicle and the duration of the phase of dominance varies (Morishita *et al.*, 1979). The event 'ovulation' marks the end of this phase and is associated with a rise in progesterone which terminates the changes observed in the mucus and renders the cervix impassable to sperm.

In practice, all that can be reliably deduced from monitoring the changes in cervical mucus is that, whilst the mucus is still showing pre-ovulatory characteristics, ovulation has not yet occurred (and could be anywhere between 12 and 96 hours away) but that once the mucus has changed, ovulation is imminent or has taken place (Nulsen *et al.*, 1987) and it is already too late for effective donor insemination (the reproductive tract no longer being readily penetrable to sperm).

Measurement of follicle volume

The recent introduction of vaginal ultrasound probes has meant that this approach can be considered as a simple alternative to mucus assessment (Vermesh *et al.*, 1987). Daily vaginal ultrasound scanning is marginally less disruptive for the patient, and the monitoring can still be performed by the donor insemination personnel, although the capital cost of the equipment is high. However, it is doubtful whether the information obtained is any more predictive than mucus assessment. There is considerable variation in the size of the dominant follicle at ovulation, both between cycles and between individuals. The size of the follicle alone is not predictive and information about its disappearance comes too late to be of value in optimally timing the insemination. This is particularly true of once daily scans where ovulation may have occurred up to 24 hours earlier.

Determination of oestradiol : progesterone ratio

Measurement of circulating oestradiol concentrations alone would confer no greater advantage than assessment of cervical mucus or determination of the size of the dominant follicle as it is related to both these parameters. Similarly, measurement of progesterone alone would give the same information as a BBT. A novel approach that has been proposed is a method to measure the concentrations of both oestradiol and progesterone (in urine as their steroid glucuronides) and to estimate their ratio (Lenton *et al.*, 1989). In this way the impact of the fall in oestradiol and the rise in progesterone following the start of the LH surge will be amplified and can, in theory, be utilized to predict imminent ovulation. In practice, available methods for assaying the steroid glucuronides are insufficiently precise, and are excessively sensitive to external factors such as the time of day when the urine sample was collected or whether the subject was taking clomiphene, to be valuable in a donor insemination programme. Methods such as this currently require laboratory facilities, and, although future technical developments may enable a semiquantitative version of the assay to be developed, it is likely that this would be more suitable for fertility control than for prediction of ovulation.

Direct predictors of ovulation

There is only one method of determining 'ovulation' directly and that is by frequent (every four hours) serial ultrasound scanning to demonstrate the disappearance of the follicle. Even with the use of a vaginal ultrasound probe, this approach is not likely to be acceptable or cost-effective as a method of monitoring for donor insemination and, in any case, is still providing information about ovulation after it has happened (albeit with much greater precision than with daily ultrasound scanning).

As has been described already (see Fig. 7.1), ovulation follows development of a mature dominant follicle (characterized by high oestradiol secretion) and occurs in direct response to a pituitary signal in the form of a surge of luteinizing hormone (LH). The LH surge is not itself a direct marker of follicular rupture but it does define an event that precedes ovulation by a fairly tightly defined time interval (Knee *et al.*, 1985). In addition, it is relatively easy to measure LH in either urine or plasma, and so monitoring of changes in LH concentrations from day to day constitutes the best method currently available for timing donor insemination.

Methods of measuring LH

There is a wide range of products available for measuring LH concentrations in either plasma or urine. Some of these products are semiquantitative (e.g. LH dipsticks) (Knee *et al.*, 1985) whilst others are fully quantitative immunoassays. The advantages with respect to precision and

Table 7.1. *Direct and indirect methods of monitoring ovulation*

Method	Limitations	Predictive power
Direct: 4 hourly ultrasound scanning	Expensive and inconvenient. May give information too late as it is probable that cervical mucus is not as receptive to spermatozoa by the time of follicular rupture.	Poor
Indirect: Basal body temperature	Cheap and easy but inaccurate.	Negligible
Cervical mucus assessment	Inexpensive but imprecise. Will result in many unnecessary inseminations and will fail to predict ovulation in some subjects.	Moderate
Daily oestradiol measurement	More precise than mucus assessment and may be difficult to interpret. No direct link with ovulation.	Poor
Daily ultrasound scanning	As expensive as oestradiol measurement and as disruptive for the patient as mucus assessment.	Poor
Daily LH measurement	Most accurate of indirect ovulation predictors but may only give a few hours warning of insemination time. No more expensive than oestradiol assay.	Good

accuracy of the fully quantitative systems mean that these are the methods of choice where limited laboratory facilities are available, but reasonable results can be obtained in most cases with the semi-quantitative products available from chemists (Bieglmayer *et al.*, 1990; Federman *et al.*, 1990). No attempt will be made to review this range as it is a rapidly expanding area and products are constantly being improved (Corsan *et al.*, 1990). Of the fully quantitative systems, the one used most extensively by the author is the ELISA from Serono Diagnostics Ltd. (Woking, Surrey). This system is fast (results available in 90 min), precise (intra- and inter-assay coefficients of 3 to 6%), has a wide operating range (0.8 to 200 U/l) and is very simple to perform requiring only a small optical density monitor. The system can measure urine and plasma in the same assay and is reasonably priced at about £1.00 sterling per determination.

Table 7.2. *Distribution of the day of onset of the LH surge in 250 regularly cycling women attending from Day 8 or 9 of the cycle for daily LH monitoring*

Day of cycle	Number of subjects	% starting LH rise	Cumulative %
<9	13	5.2	5.2
10	26	10.4	15.6
11	41	16.4	32.0
12	45	18.0	50.0
13	39	15.6	65.6
14	27	10.8	76.4
15	23	9.2	85.6
16	21	8.4	94.0
17	1	0.4	94.4
18	7	2.8	97.2
19	6	2.4	99.6
20	1	0.4	100.0

The day of maximum LH concentrations

It has been shown that, although the LH peak occurs most frequently on cycle Day 13 (counting the first day of menstrual bleeding as Day 1) the 95% confidence interval is much wider at 9 to 21 days (Lenton *et al.*, 1984). Furthermore, there is an association of follicular phase length with the woman's age with cycles progressively shortening as the woman becomes older. This means that follicular phases of 5, 6, 7 and 8 days are sometimes recorded, although it is doubtful if cycles as short as this are of normal fertility. In a recent analysis of 250 patients attending an IVF clinic for LH monitoring, it was observed that the day of onset of the LH surge was on, or before, Day 12 in 50% (Table 7.2). Note that the day of onset of the LH rise is not necessarily synonymous with the day of the LH peak and, in fact, is generally the day before the LH peak. It is, however, a more useful parameter because it identifies the first rise in LH and thus gives a longer warning of the time to ovulation and therefore to donor insemination.

Reproducibility of day of LH surge onset

If LH monitoring is to be used to time donor insemination in repeat menstrual cycles, it becomes important to know the extent of the variability in the day of maximum LH detection in successive menstrual cycles from the same woman. If this variability was strictly limited, it might be possible to detect the day of the LH surge onset in the first treatment cycle, and to carry out inseminations on equivalent days in successive cycles without further monitoring. Although Lenton and colleagues (Lenton *et al.*, 1983) have shown that there is significantly less variation in this parameter within a woman than between women, this does not mean that the LH surge will start on the same day in each menstrual cycle. In fact, data from a recent study performed to assess this variability in 20 subjects monitored for four or five cycles each showed that, whilst some subjects demonstrated a great deal more variability than others (Fig. 7.2), for all subjects the cycle-to-cycle variability was too great to allow accurate timing of donor insemination without direct monitoring.

The relationship between LH surge onset and ovulation

Although it has been known for many years that ovulation occurs about 24 h after the LH peak (Lenton *et al.*, 1983) this information is too vague to be used to individualize the timing of donor insemination.

However, a recent report from this department (Chauhan, Lenton & Barratt, in preparation) using the same serozyme LH monitoring system and 4-hourly ultrasound scanning to detect follicular rupture, has shown that the median time to ovulation was 41.5 hours from the onset of the LH surge as defined below. The 95% confidence interval was 39.8 to 45.2 hours (See Fig. 7.3).

Detection of the onset of the LH surge

It is possible for the LH surge to commence at any time of the day or night although the majority of LH surges actually begin between midnight and 0800 h. If a blood sample is collected between 0800 and 0930 h each day, the concentration of LH in the sample on the day when the first elevation over follicular phase levels is detected will give an indication of when that surge actually began. For example, if the LH concentration was 10 U/l then the surge would have only just begun; if, however, the concentration was 45 U/l, that would denote a surge that had been under way for some hours. Since the relationship between the onset of the LH surge and follicular rupture is reasonably constant, ovulation will obviously occur sooner in the woman whose LH is 45 U/l than in the woman whose LH was only 10 U/l. It is possible to derive approximate times for the event of

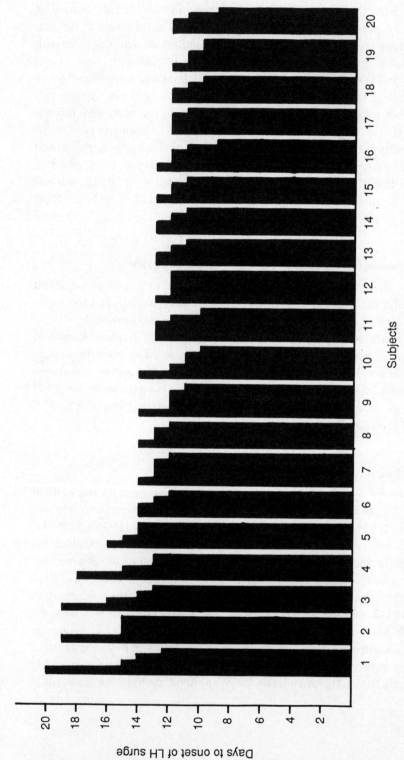

Fig. 7.2. Variation in the day of the cycle on which the spontaneous LH surge occurred in 4/5 cycles from each of 20 regularly cycling women. The vertical bars represent consecutive follicular phase lengths in each of the subjects. Although some subjects showed considerable variation (particularly subjects 1 to 5), others were consistent to within 2/3 days between cycles.

% unruptured follicles

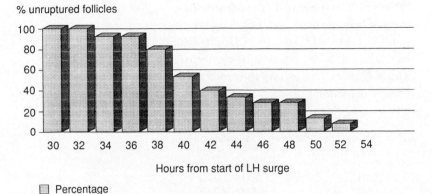

Hours from start of LH surge

☐ Percentage

Fig. 7.3. The proportion of follicles remaining intact (determined by 4-hourly ultrasound scanning), relative to the start of the spontaneous LH surge in women undergoing timed donor insemination.

ovulation relative to the onset of LH surge, and the data given in Table 7.3 demonstrates how this works in practice.

It must be stressed, however, that these LH concentration ranges relate only to the LH assay system used by the author and cannot be assumed to hold true for other assay systems without extensive confirmatory trials.

Management of LH monitoring in a DI clinic

It is important that patients should attend the clinic daily between 0800 and 0900 h from Day 9 of their cycle. In certain instances, it may be appropriate for a patient to start slightly earlier than this, if they are known to have short (<24 days) cycles.

The time 0800 to 0900 h is important for two reasons: first, because the data shown in Table 7.3 have been constructed around the pattern of LH observed at these times of day and cannot be extrapolated for use with blood samples collected at other times; and secondly, for donor insemination to be timed optimally, it will be necessary for some patients to return the same day for insemination. This means that the LH determinations should be performed as rapidly as possible so that the results are available by mid-morning. For the purposes of donor insemination, interpretation of the results is relatively straightforward. If the LH concentration is between 10 and 30 U/l, insemination should be planned

Table 7.3. *The range of LH concentrations
detected between 0800 and 0930 h on the day
of the first detectable rise (i.e. LH >10 U/l)
over follicular phase levels using the serozyme LH assay system, and the predicted
times of ovulation*

LH concentration at 0800 h	Time of ovulation (following day)
10–20 (U/l)	1800–2200 h
20–30 (U/l)	1600–2000 h
30–50 (U/l)	0900–1600 h
50–70 (U/l)	0100–0800 h

for as early as possible the following morning, but, if the LH concentration is greater than 30 U/l (and the previous day's blood sample definitely less than 10 U/l), insemination should be carried out later the same day. This means that all patients should be readily contactable at about the time the LH results become available.

Although it might seem preferable to perform LH monitoring using urine samples, which can often be analysed in the same assay as plasma samples, it should be remembered that urine LH concentrations are more variable both within and between women and so the accuracy of ovulation prediction will be somewhat reduced. Moreover, the number of cycles which cannot be interpreted will be significantly greater with urine monitoring. The reasons for the lower accuracy of urine measurements are fairly obvious and relate primarily to variations in urine output, both overnight and in response to fluid intake during the day.

Thus, although it is possible to monitor LH in urine in most patients, many of the advantages of precise timing of donor insemination will be lost, and success rates may not, in fact, be much higher than with older methods such as daily mucus assessment (Barratt *et al.*, 1989).

Atypical LH profiles

Many of the patients attending a donor insemination clinic will have perfectly normal patterns of follicular growth associated with LH concentrations that are quite familiar. However, a few patients will demonstrate endocrine abnormalities which may be associated with either high or low circulating LH concentrations and perhaps even anovulation.

References

Barratt, C. L. R., Cooke, S., Chauhan, M. & Cooke, I. D. (1989). A prospective randomized controlled trial comparing urinary LH dipsticks and basal body temperature charts to time donor insemination. *Fertility and Sterility*, **52**, 394.

Bieglmayer, C. Fischl, F. & Janisch, H. (1990). Evaluation of a simple and fast self-test for urinary luteinizing hormone. *Fertility and Sterility*, **53**, 842–6.

Corsan, G. H., Chazi, D. & Kemmann, E. (1990). Home urinary luteinizing hormone immunoassays: clinical applications. *Fertility and Sterility*, **53**, 591–601.

Federman, C. A., Dumesic, D. A., Boone, W. R. & Shapiro, S. S. (1990). Relative efficiency of therapeutic donor insemination using a luteinizing hormone monitor. *Fertility and Sterility*, **54**, 489–92.

Insler, V., Melamed, H. & Eichenbrenner, I. (1972). The cervical score: a simple semi-quantitative method for monitoring menstrual cycle. *International Journal of Gynecology and Obstetrics*, **10**, 233.

Knee, G. R., Feinman, M. A., Strauss, J. F., Blasco, L. & Goodman, D. B. P. (1985). Detection of the ovulatory luteinizing hormone (LH) surge with a semiquantitative urinary LH assay. *Fertility and Sterility*, **44**, 707–9.

Kovacs, G., Baker, H. W. G., Burger, H., DeKretser, D, Lording, D. & Lee, J. (1988). Artificial insemination with cryopreserved semen: a decade of experience. *British Journal of Obstetrics and Gynaecology*, **95**, 354–60.

Leader, A., Wiseman, D. & Taylor, P. J. (1985). The prediction of ovulation: comparison of the basal body temperature graph, cervical mucus score, and real-time pelvic ultrasonography. *Fertility and Sterility*, **43**, 385–8.

Lenton, E. A., King, H., Johnson, J. & Amos, S. (1989). Assessment of a dual *analyte* enzyme linked immunosorbent assay for urinary oestrone-3-glucuronide and pregnanediol-3-glucuronide. *Human Reproduction*, **4**, 378–80.

Lenton, E. A., Landgren, B-M., Sexton, L. & Harper, R. (1984). Normal variation in the length of the follicular phase of the menstrual cycle: effect of chronological age. *British Journal of Obstetrics and Gynaecology*, **91**, 681–4.

Lenton, E. A., Lawrence, G. F., Coleman, R. A. & Cooke, I. D. (1983). Individual variation in gonadotrophin and steroid concentrations and in lengths of follicular and luteal phases in women with regular menstrual cycles. *Clinical Reproduction and Fertility*, **2**, 143–50.

Lenton, E. A., Weston, G., Cooke, I. D. (1977). Problems in using basal body temperature recordings in an infertility clinic. *British Medical Journal*, **1**, 803–5.

Morishita, H., Hashimoto, T., Mitani, H., Tanaka, T., Higuchi, K. & Ozasa, T. (1979). Cervical mucus and prediction of the time of ovulation. *Gynecological and Obstetric Investigations*, **10**, 157–62.

Nulsen, J., Wheeler, C., Ausmanas, M. & Blasco, L. (1987). Cervical mucus changes in relationship to urinary luteinizing hormone. *Fertility and Sterility*, **48**, 783–6.

Partenteau-Carreau, S. (1981). The sympto-thermal methods. *International Journal of Fertility*, **26**, 170–81.

Quagliarello, J. & Arny, M. (1986). Inaccuracy of basal body temperature
  charts in predicting urinary luteinizing hormone surges. *Fertility and
  Sterility*, **45**, 334–7.
Richter, M. A., Haning, R. V. & Shapiro, S. S. (1984). Artificial donor
  insemination: fresh versus frozen semen: the patient as her own control.
  Fertility and Sterility, **41**, 277–80.
Smith, K. D., Rodriquez-Rigau, L. J. & Steinberger, E. (1981). The influence
  of ovulatory dysfunction and timing of insemination on the success of
  artificial insemination donor (AID) with fresh or cryopreserved semen.
  Fertility and Sterility, **36**, 496–502.
Templeton, A. A., Penney, G. C. & Lees, M. M. (1982). Relation between the
  lutcinizing hormone peak, the nadir of the basal body temperature and
  cervical mucus score. *British Journal of Obstetrics and Gynaecology*, **89**,
  985–8.
Trounson, A. O., Matthews, C. D., Kovacs, G. T., Spiers, A. Steigrad, S. J.,
  Saunders, D. M., Jones, W. R. & Fuller, S. (1981). Artificial insemination
  by frozen donor semen: results of multi-centre Australian experience.
  International Journal of Andrology, **4**, 227.
Vermesh, M., Kletzky, O.A. Davajan, V. & Israel, R. (1987). Monitoring
  techniques to predict and detect ovulation. *Fertility and Sterility*, **47**,
  259–64.

8

Donor spermatozoa and its use in assisted reproduction (IVF, GIFT)

J. C. OSBORN, C. A. YATES and G. T. KOVACS

Introduction

Donor insemination (DI) has been used for many years to overcome infertility caused by severe oligozoospermia or azoospermia. Although various factors affect the fertility of DI recipients (for an up-to-date review, see Barratt, Chauhan & Cooke, 1990), the average cumulative conception rate is approximately 55% after 6 cycles and 72% after 12 cycles of treatment (Edvinsson et al., 1990; Kovacs et al., 1988). In addition, it has been shown that more than 95% of DI pregnancies occur during the first 12 cycles of treatment (Chong & Taymor, 1975; Kovacs et al., 1988; Edvinsson et al., 1990) and the chances of conception after 12 cycles are significantly reduced (Kovacs et al., 1988; Edvinsson et al., 1990). The reason these patients fail to conceive remains to be established. However, some of the parameters must include previously undiagnosed anomalies in the ovulatory mechanism and defects in tubal function such as oocyte pick-up and gamete transport.

Until recently, failed DI couples have had the choice of either undergoing further cycles of DI, adoption or accepting their inability to have children. However, the development and application of other assisted reproduction techniques such as *in vitro* fertilization and embryo transfer (IVF-ET) or gamete intra-fallopian transfer (GIFT) has provided alternative mechanisms for overcoming those unidentified factors mentioned above. Both of these methods result in a statistically significant increase in the expectation of pregnancy compared with further cycles of DI (Cefalu et al., 1988; Federation CECOS, Lannou & Lansac, 1989; Kovacs et al., 1989; Formigli et al., 1990) and are therefore preferable despite the increased cost and inconvenience.

111

In this paper, the use of donor spermatozoa in assisted reproduction will be considered (IVF-ET, GIFT) and recent data generated from couples attending the Infertility Medical Centre in Melbourne will be used to examine 1) the methods and efficacy of sperm preparation; 2) the fertilizing ability of cryopreserved donor sperm *in vitro*; 3) the factors influencing IVF and GIFT success rates when using cryopreserved sperm and 4) the outcome of IVF and GIFT pregnancies following the use of donor semen.

Sperm preparation

In 1989, the Reproductive Technology Accreditation Committee (RTAC) of the Fertility Society of Australia issued guidelines regarding the quarantining of semen for DI which are now mandatory in all IVF units using donor semen (Appendix 1). In the author's clinic, the use of fresh donor semen was discontinued several years before the RTAC guidelines and only cryopreserved semen has been used in the IVF and GIFT program. The problems associated with the cryopreservation and thawing of human spermatozoa are well known and are discussed in detail elsewhere (Chapter 6.) Of particular relevance to the preparation of sperm for IVF and GIFT is the reduction in the number of motile sperm after cryopreservation (Keel, Webster & Roberts, 1987). For fresh semen samples from normozoospermic men, the simplest and most effective method of separating motile from non-motile sperm is the centrifugation–migration ('swim up') method (See Yates *et al.*, 1989). Briefly, an aliquot of semen is washed with culture medium, centrifuged, and the resulting pellet resuspended in a small volume of medium. Fresh medium is layered over the resuspended pellet and, after 45–60 minutes' incubation at 37 °C, the uppermost portion of the medium containing the most motile sperm is removed. A variation of the swim-up technique is to add a density medium, Ficoll (Pharmacia, Sweden) to the resuspended sperm pellet creating an interface which allows only actively motile sperm to pass across it (Cummins & Breen, 1984). However, although the centrifugation–migration techniques are the obvious and simplest methods for normal fresh semen samples, the recovery rates of motile sperm after thawing are often unsatisfactory. This is due not only to the decreased numbers of motile sperm after cryopreservation but is also related to a significant reduction in the path velocity and linearity of the surviving sperm (Chapter 6, Crittenden & Handelsman, 1990).

Table 8.1. *Comparison of pregnancy rates obtained after GIFT using cryopreserved donor sperm prepared by the centrifugation–migration or Percoll gradient technique*

Method of sperm preparation	Number of GIFT cycles	Number and % of pregnancies
Centrifugation–migration	126	53 (42.1)[a]
Percoll gradient	40	13 (32.5)[b]

Note: a versus b, $Chi^2 = 1.2$ $P = 0.28$.

By contrast, the use of Percoll (Pharmacia, Sweden) as a migration medium significantly increases the percentage recovery of motile sperm (Berger *et al.*, 1985). Using a technique developed and described by Yates *et al.* (1989), discontinuous Percoll gradients are now used routinely for the preparation of cryopreserved donor sperm for IVF and GIFT. The method involves the layering of 1.5–2.0 ml of 45% isotonic Percoll diluted with culture medium over the same volume of 90% Percoll followed by centrifugation at 200 *g* for 15–20 minutes. The resulting pellet is diluted in culture medium, centrifuged and resuspended. This sample may be used directly or may be further centrifuged and a swim-up procedure performed. The latter often produces a higher percentage of motile sperm in the final sample. Our results (Table 8.1) show that there is no significant difference in the pregnancy rate after GIFT using sperm prepared by the swim-up method or on a Percoll gradient. However, the improvement of sperm recovery after cryopreservation using Percoll gradients has enabled the number of 0.25 ml straws thawed per treatment cycle to be reduced from 7 to 3 and miniaturization of the technique (Ord *et al.*, 1990) may allow further reductions to be made. This is an important consideration when one considers the chronic shortage of good quality donors and the problems involved in the recruitment of donors from minority ethnic groups.

Fertilizing ability of donor sperm *in vitro*
For couples undergoing IVF using fresh semen from normozoospermic partners, it is current practice to add approximately 50 000 washed and progressively motile sperm to each oocyte at 4 to 6 hours after recovery. Oocytes are then examined for fertilization between 16 to 20 hours after

insemination and only those showing normal fertilization (i.e. the presence of two pronuclei) are considered for uterine transfer or cryopreservation. Table 8.2 shows that, under these conditions, 62% of oocytes fertilize normally, while an additional 8% show polyspermic fertilization. Of the remainder, approximately 3% are activated, 3.5% are degenerate, 4% are meiotically immature and 20% have reached meiotic maturity but are unfertilized. It is likely that many of the latter were still immature at the time of insemination and it has been shown that these oocytes are incapable of normal fertilization (Tesarik, Pilka & Travnik, 1988).

When oocytes are inseminated with cryopreserved sperm and checked for fertilization, there is no significant difference in the frequency distribution of oocytes displaying normal or abnormal fertilization compared with fresh sperm (Table 8.2). Moreover, increasing the number of cryopreserved sperm added from 50 000 to either 100 000 or 150 000 per oocyte, does not alter the proportion of normally fertilized oocytes but may be associated with a slight but non-significant increase in the incidence of polyspermic fertilization. Similarly, there is no difference in the numbers of normally fertilized oocytes obtained when cryopreserved sperm are prepared using either the swim-up or Percoll gradient techniques (54.8 versus 57.3% respectively) or when supernumerary oocytes are inseminated after GIFT (211/378; 55.8%). It is evident therefore, that there is no difference between the fertilizing ability of fresh and cryopreserved sperm *in vitro*. (Mahadevan *et al.*, 1983; Cohen *et al.*, 1985, Morshedi *et al.*, 1990).

Factors affecting treatment success

GIFT

Although many studies have documented the efficacy of GIFT in the treatment of infertile couples in whom the female partner has at least one patent fallopian tube (see Craft & Brinsden, 1989; Jansen *et al.*, 1990), little has been reported on the use of GIFT as an alternative treatment for couples who fail to conceive after DI. Recently, Cefalu *et al.* (1988) and Formigli *et al.* (1990) have demonstrated pregnancy rates of 52–56% in this group of patients after a single GIFT procedure. However, although their results do indeed show the value of GIFT in the treatment of failed DI patients, they were obtained using fresh donor semen. By contrast, frozen semen has always been used in the GIFT–DI programme and, as

Table 8.2. *Comparison of fertilization rate in vitro using either fresh semen from normozoospermic men or cryopreserved donor semen*

Spermatozoa used for insemination	Number of motile sperm added ($\times 10^{-3}$)	Number of oocytes inseminated	% showing normal fertilization	% multi-pronuclear	% activated	% unfertilized		
						mature	immature	degenerate
Normal (fresh)	50	688	62.1	7.9	3.2	19.5	3.9	3.5
Donor (frozen)	50	140	55.7	6.4	2.9	22.1	2.9	10.0
	100	126	58.7	11.9	3.2	14.3	9.5	2.4
	150	214	55.1	12.2	2.4	22.0	5.6	2.8
Donor (frozen)	Total	480	56.3	10.4	2.7	20.0	5.8	4.8

Table 8.3. *Comparison, on a yearly basis, of the prevalence and success rates of GIFT using donor sperm in couples with at least 12 failed DI cycles*

Year	Total number of GIFT cycles	Number and % of GIFT cycles using donor sperm (GIFT–DI)	Number and % of pregnancies after GIFT–DI
1986	40	3 (7.5)	1 (33.3)
1987	88	17 (19.3)	5 (29.4)
1988	273	62 (22.7)[a]	25 (40.3)
1989	380	56 (14.7)[b]	23 (41.1)
1990	131	17 (13.0)[c]	8 (47.1)
Total	912	155 (17.0)	62 (40.0)

Note: *a* versus *b* : $Chi^2 = 6.82$ P = 0.009.
        a versus *c* : $Chi^2 = 5.33$ P = 0.02.

shown in Table 8.3, an overall pregnancy rate of 40% has been achieved. It is of interest to note that the proportion of GIFTs using donor sperm increased from 7.5% in 1986 to a maximum of 23% in 1988 but fell significantly in 1989 and 1990. This is largely attributable to the inclusion, over the past 2 years, of more patients with mild tubal pathology and subnormal sperm parameters on the GIFT programme but also reflects an increasing use of microinjection for men with severe oligoasthenozoospermia.

The pregnancy rate obtained after GIFT–DI has also been analysed according to the age and aetiology of the infertility in the female partner. As expected, female fertility decreased significantly after 40 (Table 8.4) and, although the highest pregnancy rate is in the youngest group, there was no significant difference among the three age groups examined. Similarly, there was no difference in the pregnancy rates after GIFT between failed DI patients with no female factors and those with either endometriosis, mild tubal pathology, ovulatory defects or a combination of factors (Table 8.5). By contrast, there is a lower but not significantly different pregnancy rate in 15 couples having GIFT–DI without any previous DI treatment (26.7 versus 40%). The reason for this difference may be that the male partners were not azoospermic in these couples but showed one or more semen abnormalities. Several studies have shown that pregnancy rates are significantly higher in DI recipients with azoospermic partners when compared with those with subfertile partners

Table 8.4. *Influence of age on pregnancy rate after GIFT–DI*

Age range (years)	Mean age (years)	Number of GIFT–DI cycles	Number and % of pregnancies
25–29	28.1	34	17 (50.0)[a]
30–34	32.1	77	30 (39.0)[a]
35–39	37.0	52	19 (36.5)[a]
≥40	41.7	7	0 (0)[b]
Total	33.2	170	66 (38.8)

Note: Different superscripts indicate significant difference: $P < 0.05$.
GIFT is only performed on DI patients who have had a minimum of 12 failed DI cycles.

Table 8.5. *Outcome of GIFT procedure with donor sperm in relation to female aetiology in couples with failed DI*

Female aetiology	Number of GIFT–DI cycles	Number and % of pregnancies
Idiopathic	91	37 (40.7)
Endometriosis	19	7 (36.8)
Tubal pathology	27	10 (37.0)
Ovulatory defects	5	1 (20.0)
Combined factors	9	4 (44.4)
Total	155	62 (40.0)

Note: GIFT is only performed on DI patients who have had a minimum of 12 failed DI cycles.

Table 8.6. *Life table analysis of pregnancy rates per GIFT–DI cycle in couples with failed DI*

Cycle Number	Number of GIFT–DI cycles	Number of pregnancies	Pregnancy rate per cycle (%)	Cumulative pregnancy rate (%)
1	109	44	40.4	40.4 ± 3.6
2	31	14	45.2	67.3 ± 4.8
3	10	1	10.0	70.6 ± 7.8
4	5	3	60.0	88.2 ± 5.0

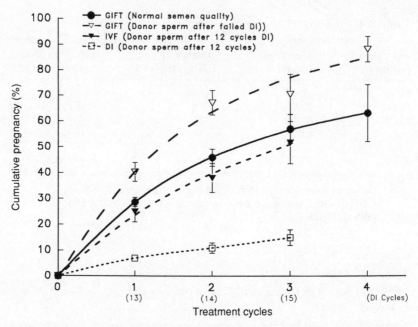

Fig. 8.1. Cumulative pregnancy rates per cycle (mean + SEM) for GIFT, IVF and DI, each using donor sperm after 12 or more failed cycles of DI compared with the cumulative conception rate for GIFT using normal semen quality.

(see Barratt *et al.*, 1990) and it is therefore likely that the fertility of women undergoing GIFT–DI will be higher in those with azoospermic partners.

The outcome of GIFT–DI was assessed using life-table methods (Kovacs *et al.*, 1986) to calculate cumulative pregnancy rates and by applying a mathematical model of cumulative pregnancy (Guzick & Rock, 1981; Guzick, Bross & Rock, 1982) to estimate clinically pertinent data. This regression model expresses the cumulative pregnancy rate after n cycles (P_n) in terms of two clinically meaningful parameters: $P_n = c(1 - e^{\lambda n})$ where c is the 'cure rate' or proportion of patients who will conceive if sufficient numbers of GIFT–DI cycles are performed and λ is the probability of pregnancy per cycle among those cured and n is the number of cycles. From life-table analysis (Table 8.6), it is calculated that 40.4% of patients will conceive after one cycle of GIFT–DI and that 88.2% would conceive after four cycles. This compares with an estimated 63% pregnancy rate after four cycles of GIFT in normozoospermic couples (Fig. 8.1) and a pregnancy rate of between 40 and 45% after four cycles of DI (Kovacs *et al.*, 1989; Edvinsson *et al.*, 1990). The maximum likelihood estimates of the 'cure rate' (c) and the probability of pregnancy per GIFT–DI cycle among the cured (λ) are 0.95 and 0.55 respectively, showing that GIFT–DI will ultimately result in close to a 100% pregnancy rate. However, corresponding estimates for normozoospermic couples undergoing GIFT are 0.73 and 0.50 suggesting that there is a lower likelihood of pregnancy in this group of patients. Nevertheless, a comparison of the cumulative pregnancy rates observed after GIFT–DI with those after cycles 13 to 16 of DI (Fig. 8.1) clearly shows that the chances of pregnancy after GIFT are significantly higher. Thus GIFT with cryopreserved donor semen is an effective procedure after failed DI.

IVF

Prior to the advent of GIFT at the end of 1984 (Asch *et al.*, 1984), it was the policy of this unit to offer IVF to couples with failed DI. In an analysis of results from 1980 to 1986, Kovacs *et al.* (1989) showed conclusively that the chance of success by IVF after 12 failed cycles of DI was significantly higher than for further cycles of DI. These differences are illustrated graphically in Fig. 8.1. The cumulative pregnancy curve for patients undergoing IVF with donor insemination (IVF–DI) after failed DI is significantly lower than that of women having GIFT–DI with a 'cure rate' and probability of pregnancy per cycle in the former of 0.76 and 0.37 respectively. (The probability values comparing pregnancy rates after IVF–DI and GIFT–DI are: after 1 cycle <0.05; 2 cycles <0.005, 3 cycles <0.01.) It is therefore evident that GIFT should be the method of choice for those failed DI couples in whom the female partner has at least one patent fallopian tube. Moreover, with a cumulative conception rate of approximately 88% after four cycles of GIFT–DI treatment (Fig. 8.1), it is clear that, as in normal DI therapy, success is dependent upon couples returning for further treatment.

It is important then to ask the question when should IVF with donor sperm be performed? An analysis of the aetiology of women undergoing 59 cycles of IVF with donor sperm after failed DI over the past 18 months (Table 8.7) shows that only 34 (58%) had tubal disease or pelvic adhesions, whereas 25 (42%) had ostensibly normal tubes and were, in fact, suitable for GIFT. Indeed, six of these patients had either GIFT or tubal embryo stage transfer (TEST) in subsequent treatment cycles and two conceived. Moreover, while 91% of the GIFT–DI cycles had previously had failed DI, 26% of the IVF–DI cycles were associated with

Table 8.7. *Outcome of IVF cycles with donor sperm in couples with and without previous failed DI cycles and in the presence or absence of tubal disease*

Previous failed DI[*]	Tubal pathology	Number of cycles	Number of embryo transfers	Number and % of pregnancies
Yes	Yes	34	32	10 (31.3)[a]
Yes	No	25	22	1 (4.6)[b]
No	Yes	15	15	2 (13.3)
No	No	7	6	0 (0.0)
Total	—	81	75	13 (17.3)

Note: a versus b: $Chi^2 = 5.73$ $P = 0.02$.
[*] Minimum 12 failed DI cycles.

semen abnormalities but had not had DI therapy. In the majority of these cases (20/22; 91%), the use of donor sperm resulted from the failure on one or more occasions of the male partner's sperm to fertilize oocytes *in vitro*. By contrast, in the other two cycles, donor sperm was used following the failure of a quadraplegic patient to produce a semen sample. As in the IVF–DI cycles after failed DI, a significant proportion (7/22; 31%) of patients undergoing IVF–DI after failed IVF with partner's sperm did not have any tubal pathology. Interestingly, there is a difference in pregnancy rate after IVF–ET between those women with and without tubal disease which reaches significance (Table 8.7; $P < 0.02$) in the failed DI group. However, this difference is probably illusory since 12 of the failed DI cycles in women with normal tubes were accounted for by just three women, two of whom were over 40 and the other had poor oocytes which showed supranormal levels of polyspermy.

It is clear that the major deciding factor for IVF or GIFT is the presence or absence of infertility factors in the female partner. There is no doubt that several tubal disease and/or pelvic adhesions necessitate IVF and embryo transfer. However, it has been clearly shown that there is no difference in pregnancy rates after GIFT using donor sperm in women with either endometriosis, mild tubal pathology, or ovulatory defects compared to those with no discernible factors (Table 8.5). There is, therefore, no logical reason for using IVF in these patients except perhaps when large numbers of supernumerary oocytes fail to fertilize. Under these circumstances, the probability of pregnancy after GIFT is significantly decreased (Cushnahan & Osborn, 1991) and it may be necessary to confirm fertilization *in vitro* before undertaking further GIFT cycles. Nevertheless, any embryos resulting from IVF should be replaced using the TEST procedure into the more beneficial environment of the fallopian tubes rather than into the uterus (Yovich *et al.*, 1988).

In the IVF and GIFT program, cryopreserved donor semen is used for those women who have failed to conceive after 12 or more cycles of DI or who, in cases of severe male factor infertility, experience failed fertilization *in vitro*. More recently, however, Pool *et al.* (1990) have suggested that donor sperm may also be used as a 'backup' procedure for those male factor couples who initially want to inseminate all oocytes with husband's sperm and use donor sperm only if the attempt by the husband fails. Conventionally, using donor semen as a backup for husband's sperm in IVF involves either mixing both sets of sperm before insemination or inseminating some of the oocytes with husband's sperm and the rest with donor. However, preliminary evidence suggests that reinseminating with donor sperm after failed fertilization with husband's sperm produces a high fertilization rate (70%) and can result in clinical pregnancies (Pool *et al.*, 1990). This technique confirms Trounson & Webbs' (1984) original finding that the fertilization rate of oocytes reinseminated with donor sperm is significantly higher than those reinseminated with husband's sperm. However, although clinical pregnancies can occur after IVF–ET with embryos resulting from reinsemination with husband's sperm, only 1 to 2% of the embryos implant (Pampiglione *et al.*, 1990). In Pool *et al*'s (1990) study, the zygotes produced by 'donor rescue' were transferred into the fallopian tubes (zygote intrafallopian transfer: ZIFT) in only four couples with two clinical pregnancies. Thus on the basis of these results, it is perhaps premature to conclude that 'donor rescue' and ZIFT is an effective treatment for male factor infertility. Nevertheless, if further studies do establish the validity of this technique, then 'donor rescue' may indeed be an important development in the use of donor semen in assisted reproduction.

Pregnancy outcome

From 1979 to 1988, 294 clinical pregnancies (~8% of all IVF pregnancies) were achieved following the use of IVF–DI in Australia and New Zealand (Data from the National Perinatal Statistics Unit, 1990). The outcome of these pregnancies was as follows: live births, 200, 68%; stillbirths, 12, 4.1%; spontaneous abortions, 69, 23.5%; ectopic pregnancy, 12, 4.1%

Table 8.8. *Outcome of pregnancy after GIFT with donor semen compared with outcome of all GIFT pregnancies included in the Australian and New Zealand register*

	GIFT pregnancies* (1985–1988)		GIFT–DI pregnancies (1986–1989)	
Outcome of pregnancy	Number	%	Number	%
Spontaneous abortion	338	22.8	11	22.0
Termination of pregnancy	11	0.7	0	—
Ectopic pregnancy	71	4.8	2	4.0
Stillbirth	33	2.2	0	—
Livebirth	1029	69.4	37	74.0
Total	1482	100.0	50	100.0

* Data from National Perinatal Statistics Unit (1990).

and termination of pregnancy, 1, 0.3%. The plurality of the 212 viable pregnancies was: singletons, 161, 75.9%; twins, 45, 21.2% and triplets, 6, 2.8%. The pregnancy outcome and incidence of multiple births after IVF–DI was similar to that observed in all IVF pregnancies. To date, the Australian and New Zealand register has not presented data on the outcome of pregnancies after GIFT–DI. An analysis of the 57 clinical pregnancies obtained in our clinic from 1986 to 1990 (Table 8.8) shows that of the 50 with a known outcome, 37 (74%) resulted in live births, 2 (4%) were ectopic and 11 (22%) spontaneously aborted. Of the live births, 25 (67.6%) were singletons, 11 (29.7%) were twins and 1 (2.7%) were a quadruplet delivery. These results are similar to the overall result for GIFT in the register (Table 8.8), although the prevalence of twins was higher after GIFT–DI (29.7 versus 19.7%). It is of interest to note that there is an increased risk of spontaneous abortion, ectopic and multiple pregnancy after both IVF–DI and GIFT–DI compared to routine DI treatment (cf. Edvinsson *et al.*, 1990), but that there is little difference in pregnancy outcome between these two groups.

Conclusions

In this chapter it has been shown that the use of cryopreserved donor sperm in IVF and GIFT is effective in overcoming infertility in patients failing to conceive after DI. Moreover, it is evident that the chance of success after GIFT is very much higher than that obtained with IVF. Thus after four cycles of GIFT, the cumulative pregnancy rate is nearly 90%. Although both IVF and GIFT result in a higher pregnancy rate compared with the first cycle of DI, the authors would not advocate simply replacing DI therapy with IVF–DI or GIFT–DI. The greater complexity, stress and costs involved in IVF/GIFT treatment together with the increased prevalence of spontaneous abortions and multiple pregnancy does not make this a viable option. On the other hand, only offering IVF or GIFT after 12 or more failed cycles of DI have been completed is also not cost effective. It is suggested that IVF/GIFT with donor semen be considered much earlier than is currently practised and proposed that patients with demonstrated tubal patency who fail to conceive after six cycles of DI should then undergo four cycles of GIFT. This is the case in the authors' clinic. The conception rates of DI progressively decline after six cycles such that, from cycle 7 to cycle 12, the chance of pregnancy only increases by about 15%. By contrast, a single GIFT cycle gives a 40% chance of pregnancy. Such an approach would not only maximize the chances of success but would also have a dramatic effect on the usage and availability of what is often a limited resource, namely donor semen.

References

Asch, R. H., Ellsworth, L. R., Balmaceda, J. P. & Wong, P. C. (1984). Pregnancy after translaparoscopic gamete intrafallopian transfer. *Lancet*, **ii**, 1034–5.

Barratt, C. L. R., Chauhan, M. & Cooke, I. D. (1990). Donor insemination – a look to the future. *Fertility and Sterility*, **54**, 375–87.

Berger, T., Marrs, R. P. & Moyer, D. L. (1985). Comparison of techniques for the selection of motile spermatozoa. *Fertility and Sterility*, **43**, 268–73.

Cefalu, E., Cittadini, E., Balmaceda, J. P., Guastella, G., Ord, T., Rojas, F. J. & Asch, R. H. (1988). Successful gamete intrafallopian transfer following failed artificial insemination by donor: evidence for a defect in gamete transport. *Fertility and Sterility*, **50**, 279–82.

Chong, A. P. & Taymor, M. L. (1975). Sixteen years' experience with therapeutic donor insemination. *Fertility and Sterility*, **26**, 791–6.

Cohen, J., Edwards, R. G., Fehilly, C. B., Fishel, S. B., Hewitt, J., Rowland, G. F., Steptoe, P. C., Walter, D. E. & Webster, J. (1985). *In vitro* fertilization using cryopreserved donor semen in cases where both partners are infertile. *Fertility and Sterility*, **43**, 570.

Craft, I. & Brinsden, P. (1989). Alternatives to IVF: the outcome of 1071 first GIFT procedures. *Human Reproduction*, 4 Suppl., 29–36.

Crittenden, J. A. & Handelsman, D. J. (1990) Effect of cryopreservation on sperm motion. *Proceedings of the 9th Scientific Meeting, Fertility Society of Australia*, p. 77.

Cummins, J. M. & Breen, T. M. (1984). Separation of progressively motile spermatozoa from human semen by sperm rise through a density gradient. *Australian Journal of Medical Laboratories*, **5**, 15–20.

Cushnahan, L. A. & Osborn, J. C. (1992). The *in vitro* fertilization of supernumerary oocytes in a GIFT program is predictive of pregnancy outcome. *Human Reproduction*, (In press).

Edvinsson, A., Forssman, L., Milsom, I. & Nordfors, G. (1990). Factors in the infertile couple influencing the success of artificial insemination with donor semen. *Fertility and Sterility*, **53**, 81–7.

Federation CECOS, Le Lannou, D. & Lansac, J. (1989). Artificial procreation with frozen donor semen: experience of the French Federation CECOS. *Human Reproduction*, **4**, 757–61.

Formigli, L., Coglitore, M. T., Roccio, C., Belotti, G., Stangalini, A. & Formigli, G. (1990). One-hundred-and-six gamete intra-Fallopian transfer procedures with donor semen. *Human Reproduction*, **5**, 549–52.

Guzick, D. S., Bross, D. S. & Rock, J. A. (1982). A parametric method for comparing cumulative pregnancy curves following infertility therapy. *Fertility and Sterility*, **37**, 503–7.

Guzick, D. S. & Rock, J. A. (1981). Estimation of a model of cumulative pregnancy following infertility therapy. *American Journal of Obstetrics and Gynecology*, **104**, 573–8.

Jansen, R. P. S., Anderson, J. C., Birrell, W. S. R., Lyncham, R. C., Sutherland, P. D., Turner, M., Flowers, D. & Ciancaglini, E. (1990). Outpatient gamete intrafallopian transfer: a clinical analysis of 710 cases. *Medical Journal of Australia*, **153**, 182–8.

Keel, B. A., Webster, B. W. & Roberts, D. K. (1987). Effects of cryopreservation on the motility characteristics of human spermatozoa. *Journal of Reproduction and Fertility*, **81**, 213–?.

Kovacs, G. T., Baker, G., Burger, H., de Kretser, D., Lording, D. W. & Lee, J. (1988). AID with cryopreserved semen: a decade of experience. *British Journal of Obstetrics and Gynaecology*, **95**, 354–60.

Kovacs, G. T., King, C., Rogers, P., Wood, C., Baker, H. W. G. & Yates, C. (1989). *In vitro* fertilization, a practical option after failed artificial insemination with donor semen. *Reproduction, Fertility and Development*, **1**, 383–6.

Kovacs, G. T., Rogers, P., Leeton, J. F., Trounson, A. O. & Wood, C. (1986). *In vitro* fertilization and embryo transfer – prospects of pregnancy by life-table analysis. *Medical Journal of Australia*, **144**, 682–3.

Mahadevan, M. M., Trounson, A. O. & Leeton, J. F. (1983). Successful use of human semen cryobanking for *in vitro* fertilization. *Fertility and Sterility*, **40**, 340.

Morshedi, M., Oehninger, S., Veeck, L. L., Ertunc, H., Bocca, S. & Acosta, A. A. (1990). Cryopreserved/thawed semen for *in vitro* fertilization: results from fertile donors and infertile patients. *Fertility and Sterility*, **54**, 1093–9.

National Perinatal Statistics Unit and Fertility Society of Australia. (1990). *IVF and GIFT Pregnancies, Australia and New Zealand, 1988*. Sydney: National Perinatal Statistics Unit.

Ord, T., Patrizio, P., Marello, E., Balmaceda, J. P. & Asch, R. H. (1990). Mini-Percoll: a new method of semen preparation for IVF in severe male factor infertility. *Human Reproduction*, **5**, 987–9.

Pampiglione, J. S., Mills, C., Campbell, S., Steer, C., Kingsland, C. & Mason, B. A. (1990). The clinical outcome of reinsemination of human oocytes fertilized *in vitro*. *Fertility and Sterility*, **53**, 306–10.

Pool, T. B., Martin, J. E., Ellsworth, L. R., Perez, J. B. & Atiee, S. H. (1990). Zygote intrafallopian transfer with 'donor rescue': a new option for severe male factor infertility. *Fertility and Sterility*, **54**, 166–8.

Tesarik, J., Pilka, L. & Travnik, P. (1988). Zona pellucida resistance to sperm penetration before the completion of human oocyte maturation. *Journal of Reproduction and Fertility*, **83**, 487–95.

Trounson, A. O. & Webb, J. (1984). Fertilization of human oocytes following reinsemination *in vitro*. *Fertility and Sterility*, **41**, 816–19.

Yates, C. A., Thomas, C., Kovacs, G. T. & de Kretser, D. M. (1989). Andrology, male factor infertility and IVF. In *Clinical* in vitro *fertilization*, ed. C. Wood & A. O. Trounson, pp. 95–111. Berlin: Springer-Verlag.

Yovich, J. L., Yovich, M. J. & Edirisinghe, R. W. (1988). The relative chance of pregnancy following tubal or uterine transfer procedures. *Fertility and Sterility*, **49**, 858–64.

RTAC Guideline

Appendix 1

Quarantining of semen for donor insemination

This guideline has been prepared by RTAC at the request of the directors of several IVF Units during the course of visits by RTAC to accredit programmes over the past year.

The debate is whether the period for quarantine be 3 or 6 months, since the practice seems to vary from State to State. Thus the Victorian Health AIDS Committee recommends a six month period while in New South Wales the period has been set at three months. The American Fertility Society in its guidelines [1986] proposed a 60 day quarantine period based presumably on the evidence that the vast majority of HIV infected individuals will seroconvert within 4 weeks. Since then, however, it has become apparent that in rare instances seroconversion may take up to 4 months. This information is based on up to date evidence supplied by Professor A. Basten, Chairman, AIDS Task Force.

On the basis of all available evidence RTAC recommends that the following guideline be observed in all Units that use Donor Insemination.

Every semen donor must make a lifestyle declaration, undergo HIV antibody screening and have his semen quarantined for a period of six months, when he must undergo a further HIV antibody screen.

RTAC believes that this guideline is in the best interests of both patients and staff and that the maintenance of this practice will not impose inordinate logistic difficulties in the conduct of Donor Insemination programmes.

January 30, 1989

9

The influence of female fertility on donor insemination success: possible reasons for failure

M. CHAUHAN

Introduction

Three major factors have been suggested as influencing the success and outcome of donor insemination. These include the fertilizing potential of donor semen (Mayaux *et al.*, 1985), accurate timing of inseminations (Smith *et al.*, 1981) and the potential fertility of donor insemination recipients (Barratt *et al.*, 1990; Chauhan *et al.*, 1989). A review of the literature has shown that there is a gross deficiency of good data concerning the relative importance of the latter point in determining the outcome of this treatment. This is primarily because donor insemination (DI) represents a solution for male infertility/subfertility, and hence it has been wrongly assumed that correction of this factor will normalize the 'fertility of the couple'. The female partner has often been considered to be of 'normal fertility' and therefore minimally investigated (to elicit factors which may impair her potential fertility) prior to the commencement of the treatment. The importance of female fertility in determining the success of donor insemination is obvious – the higher the fertility of the female partner the less time will be required to achieve a conception. This chapter will aim to discuss the relative importance of factors which may influence female fertility. This will enable clinicians practising insemination by donor to detect couples with good and poor prognosis, and hence to provide prognostic guidelines as to the likely outcome of the treatment.

Fertility has been defined as the 'capacity of the woman to bear children'. The degree of 'potential fertility' has been quantified in many ways. One such method has been by calculating the probability of conception per month (monthly conception rate) i.e. the 'fecundability'. The higher the fecundability the more fertile the woman, and the lower the fecundability the lower the fertility. Fecundability and cumulative conception curves will be used in this chapter to assess the effect of infertility factors on the fertility of donor insemination recipients.

The *'natural potential fertility or fecundability'* of the female partner is difficult to estimate since in the present general population complex social and cultural factors and voluntary contraception are utilized to control fertility. Some studies have, however, assessed the natural fertility of communities in which the use of voluntary contraception is banned and in which there are no economic factors to limit the family size. One such community is the Hutterites. These are a Protestant sect living in farming communes in the United States. They have mono-gamous relationships in which the use of contraception and abortion is against their religious principles. A study by Eaton and Mayer (1953) showed that the peak fertility of these women occurred at the age of 22 (70% live birth rate). From these data it was also estimated that the total fertility of these women, i.e. the expected number of children during the reproductive life span would be 10.9.

Such a high level of fertility is unlikely in a present-day population. This is because the use of voluntary contraception (such as the oral contraceptive pill, intrauterine contraceptive device), increase in sexual promiscuity leading to a higher incidence of pelvic inflammatory disease and tubal damage and social/financial pressures are all working to control potential fertility. The overall potential fertility of a United Kingdom population has been estimated by Cooke *et al.* (1981). These authors estimated the monthly fecundability using the data of Vessey *et al.* (1978). Vessey and colleagues calculated the rate of outcome of pregnancy in parous women after stopping barrier contraception. They reported a cumulative conception rate of 54% after 6 months which rose to 82% after 1 year and plateaued to 95% after 2 years. Cooke *et al.* (1981) estimated a fecundability of 0.12 for this population. Similarly, Westoff *et al.* (1961) have estimated a fecundability of 0.20 for the United States of America. These fecundability rates are an average for the general population. Such a population would contain women of very high fertility, those with average fertility and those with low fertility. These findings can be expressed in a different way. With a fecundability rate of 0.12, it would be expected that the mean number of months required to achieve a conception would be 8 and, with a fecundability rate of 0.20, the mean number of months required to achieve a conception would be 5.

Keeping this data in mind the discussion in this chapter will aim:

1. to assess the fecundability of a donor insemination population;
2. to assess effects of infertility factors on the fertility of DI recipients.

Factors affecting the potential fertility of DI recipients

Semen abnormality of the partner

It has been shown repeatedly that the fertility of donor insemination recipients varies in relation to the presence or absence of sperms in the semen of their partners. Donor insemination recipients whose partners are sterile (azoospermic) have significantly higher fertility than those whose partners are subfertile, i.e. have varying degress of semen abnormalities such as oligozoospermia, asthenozoospermia and teratozoospermia (subfertile). The reason for this is that DI recipients whose partners are azoospermic represent an unselected group of women containing those with high, average and low fertility while those women with subfertile partners represent a selected subgroup from which the highly fertile females have been excluded through spontaneous conception prior to presenting for donor insemination. In 1982, Emperaire *et al.* showed that, of 131 insemination recipients, the pregnancy rates were significantly higher in those patients with azoospermic partners (70%) when compared to those with subfertile partners (48.8%). A multicentre study from Australia involving seven donor insemination centres and 1357 patients showed that the pregnancy rates in women of azoospermic partners after 12 cycles of insemination was 63% which was significantly higher ($P < 0.01$) than those whose partners were subfertile (50%). Significantly higher cumulative conception rates and fecundability has consistently been demonstrated in DI recipients with azoospermic partners when compared to those with subfertile partners (Albrecht *et al.*, 1982; Foss & Hull, 1986; Chauhan *et al.*, 1989).

Little has been reported on the variation of female fertility in relation to other semen abnormalities such as oligozoospermia, asthenozoospermia, teratozoospermia or a combination of one or more of these factors. Kremer (1982) reported on the variation in pregnancy rates in relation to the motile sperm density of the partners of the donor insemination recipients. His findings showed that, as the motile sperm density increased, the pregnancy rates decreased. Surprisingly, in his DI recipients, the pregnancy rate was 100% after 18 cycles of insemination in those with azoospermic partners and partners with less than 2 million motile sperms in the semen. He also showed that as the number of motile sperms increased (2–9 million and greater than 10 million) the pregnancy rates decreased (from 73% to 63% respectivey). Recently we have also shown that the fertility of donor insemination recipients decreased significantly with an increase in the *number* of abnormal semen factors, i.e. oligozoospermia, asthenozoospermia, teratozoospermia of the partner of the donor insemination recipients. This study showed that those donor insemination recipients whose partners had three factor abnormalities (density, motility and morphology) had significantly ($P <$ 0.05) higher fecundability (0.06) and cumulative conception rates (70%) when compared to those DI recipients whose partners had only one factor abnormality – fecundability of 0.01 and cumulative conception rate of 20%. Those donor insemination recipients with two semen factor abnormalities (density/motility, motility/morphology or morphology/ density) had a fecundability of 0.04 which was higher than those with a single factor abnormality but the difference was not statistically significant. The author also used a Cox's proportional hazards regression model to determine which of the semen variables assessed, i.e. density, motility or morphology could best predict the potential fertility of the donor insemination recipients. The analysis showed that progressive sperm motility was the most significant factor ($P < 0.005$) in predicting the outcome and fertility of the donor insemination recipients. As the progressive sperm motility increased the conception rates decreased. The highest fecundability (0.09) in those donor insemination recipients whose partners had progressive sperm motility of less than 20% while the lowest (0.03) was in those whose partners had progressive sperm motility >20% (Chauhan & Barratt, unpublished data).

Some confirmatory evidence of the variation in female fertility in relation to their partner's semen abnormality has come from male infertility clinics. Hargreave and Elton (1985) reported variation in the fecundability of the partners of men attending a male infertility clinic. They showed that there was a gradual but significant increase in the fecundability (with natural conception) of the partners of subfertile men with an increase in the number of motile sperm. Of 955 infertile couples the fecundability in the partners of azoospermic men was 0.4% which increased to 5.9% when the partner had 10 million motile sperms/ml. Therefore one can conclude from these results that the lower the motile sperm density the lower the fertilizing potential of spermatozoa. Hence it may be inferred that if the females that did not conceive presented for donor insemination then the potential fertility of these women would decrease with an increase in the motile sperm density of their partners. Such simple semen analysis can be used to detect DI recipients with potential high and low fertility and hence provide prognostic guidelines as to the likely success.

The presence or absence of female infertility factors

Infertility factors such as endometriosis, pelvic adhesions, tubal disease, fibroids and ovulatory disorders have been shown to affect the fertility of infertile women but their role in determining the success and outcome of donor insemination has only been documented in a limited way. This is because most donor insemination centres perform limited investigations (such as confirmation of ovulation by BBT charts, tubal patency by hysterosalpingography) prior to the commencement of the treatment. More intensive investigations are usually only performed after six or more cycles of failed inseminations (Barratt, Chauhan & Cooke, 1990). Therefore the role of the above mentioned individual fertility factors in determining the fertility of the insemination recipients and to what extent they contribute to failure of donor insemination is generally unknown. Each factor will be considered and its implications for the fertility of insemination recipients discussed.

Endometriosis

The incidence of endometriosis in fertile women has been reported to be between 2.5% and 5.0% (Strathy et al., 1982). In infertile women an incidence of 6% to 50% has been reported. Williams and Pratt (1977) reported that from a prospective study of 1000 consecutive laparotomies 50% of the patients had endometriosis. In a survey of the causes of infertility, Hull et al. (1985) reported an annual incidence of 6% of couples having endometriosis as their primary disorder. The incidence of endometriosis in donor insemination recipients has not been properly documented since investigations are only performed in those that fail to conceive. Bergquist et al. (1982) reported that 13 (46%) out of 28 failed donor insemination patients who had laparoscopies had endometriosis. Emperaire et al. (1982) reported that 7% of their DI recipients had endometriosis. Gillett et al. (1986) showed that 24% of the DI recipients who failed to conceive after three or more cycles of insemination were found to have stage 1 and stage 2 endometriosis. Hammond et al. (1986) reported an incidence of 15% of DI recipients with endometriosis. Therefore the incidence quoted from DI centres is similar to that stated from general infertility clinics. Since the incidence of endometriosis is higher in those women with infertility when compared to those without fertility problems, it may be deduced that endometriosis is associated with infertility and it may be a cause of the infertility. However, it has been shown that the association between endometriosis and infertility does not have a simple cause and effect relationship. It has also been conclusively shown that the treatment of this condition does not improve the fertility of the infertile patients (Thomas & Cooke, 1987).

Many donor insemination studies have suggested that endometriosis is associated with a significant reduction in the fertility of insemination recipients and therefore contributes to the failure of donor insemination. Hammond *et al.* (1986) reported a fecundability of only 0.04 in those with mild endometriosis which was significantly lower when compared to those DI recipients without any infertility factors (fecundability of 0.20). Similarly Bordson *et al.* (1986) showed a significantly diminished fecundability of 0.07 in those with varying degrees of endometriosis (mild, moderate and severe) when compared to those without any infertility factor (0.15). Jansen (1986) demonstrated that, in seven patients with untreated grade 1 endometriosis diagnosed prior to commencement of donor insemination, a fecundability of only 0.036 after 15 cycles of insemination was significantly lower than that in those without endometriosis (0.12). Therefore there is considerable evidence that the presence of endometriosis is associated with reduced fertility of donor insemination recipients.

Does treatment of endometriosis improve the fertility and probability of conception of infertile patients? The treatment of patients in general infertility clinics has shown that treatment does not improve the fertility of these women. Seibel *et al.* (1982), have shown from a prospective study comparing conception rates in those with treated grade 1 endometriosis (treatment with Danazol) with those receiving no treatment, that there were no significant differences in the conception rates between these two groups after 12 months. In a more recent, randomized prospective double blind controlled trial assessing the effect of gestrinone versus placebo Thomas and Cooke (1987) showed that there were no significant differences in cumulative conception rates in women treated with gestrinone and those given placebo. These authors also showed that the conception rates in females with treated endometriosis were not significantly different from those with unexplained infertility. Recently we have shown that the fecundability of 37 DI recipients with grade 1 endometriosis treated prior to commencement of inseminations was 0.09 which was not significantly different from those DI recipients with no infertility factors (0.08) (Chauhan & Barratt, unpublished data). Therefore there is considerable evidence that endometriosis is associated with diminished female fertility and that treatment of minor degrees of this condition is unlikely to improve female fertility.

Ovulatory disorders

Of the factors that affect female fertility, the treatment of ovulatory disorders has been noted to have the most significant effect on the fertility of the infertile couples. The incidence of this disorder in the general infertile population has been quoted to be between 20% and 40%. Hull *et al.* (1985) reported an annual incidence of 21% from a regional infertility clinic. Collins *et al.* (1983) quoted an incidence of 30% of infertile couples having ovulatory disorders. Conception rates of 50–80% have been reported from general infertility clinics for treated ovulatory disorders secondary to hypothalamic hypopituitarism, ovarian abnormality and hyperprolactinaemia (Whitelaw *et al.*, 1970; Katayama *et al.*, 1979). Hull *et al.* (1985) have reported a cumulative conception rate of 96% after 24 months in those with ovulatory disorder secondary to hypothalamic hypopituitarism.

The incidence of ovulatory disorder in donor insemination recipients has been quoted to be between 10% and 60%. Bradshaw *et al.* (1987) reported that 40% of their DI recipients had treatment with clomiphene for ovulatory disorders while Bergquist *et al.* (1982) reported that 11% of the women in their study had ovulatory problems. Similarly Hammond *et al.* (1986) reported an incidence of 44%. As in general infertility patients, treatment has been noted to improve the fertility of the insemination recipients. Corson (1980) noted that 50% of his patients treated with clomiphene citrate conceived but the time to conception was significantly longer (5.5 cycles) than in those who ovulated spontaneously (3.3 cycles). Smith *et al.* (1981) also found that the pregnancy rates in those with treated ovulatory disorders (62.6%) were not significantly different from those ovulating spontaneously (85.7%) but the time to conception was longer in those receiving treatment (4.8 cycles) when compared to those ovulating spontaneously (2.8 cycles). Some studies have noted that although the treatment of ovulatory disorders improves the fertility of donor insemination recipients, their fertility is still significantly lower than those who ovulate spontaneously.

Hammond *et al.* (1986) reported a fecundability of 0.12 in patients with treated ovulatory dysfunction which was significantly lower than those insemination recipients with no infertility factors (fecundability of 0.20). Bradshaw *et al.* (1987) have shown that the fecundability of those ovulating spontaneously was significantly higher ($P < 0.05$) than those being treated with clomiphene citrate although there was no significant difference in the eventual cumulative conception rate between these two groups. In a recent study, Chauhan *et al.* (1989) have shown that DI recipients with ovulatory disorders have significantly lower fecundability (0.09) than those with no infertility factors and azoospermic partners (0.18). This lower fertility of DI recipients with ovulatory disorders may explain why the time to conception for those with this disorder is significantly longer than those who ovulate spontaneously.

One may conclude that the treatment of ovulatory disorders certainly improves the probability of conception but the fertility is still lower than in those without any infertility factors.

Other infertility factors

The data on the effects of other infertility factors such as tubal disease, pelvic adhesions and fibroids on the fertility of DI recipients are sparse. Studies which have suggested that these factors reduce fertility of DI recipients have done so on the basis of finding these disorders in recipients who have failed to conceive but the incidence of these factors in those that conceived was unknown. However, the causal association between these factors and infertility has been well documented from general infertility clinics. Bradshaw *et al.* (1986) showed a cumulative conception rate of 50% in 28 donor insemination recipients with unilateral tubal patency. This was significantly lower ($P < 0.05$) than those with bilaterally patent tubes (cumulative conception rate of 80%). Chauhan *et al.* (1989) have shown that the fecundability of DI recipients with more than one infertility factor, i.e. endometriosis, ovulatory disorder, tubal disease, fibroids and pelvic adhesions) was only 0.02. These authors also showed that this was significantly lower ($P < 0.005$) than those with treated endometriosis or treated ovulatory disorders – fecundability of 0.09. It is interesting to note that this latter study showed that a combination of infertility factors has a major additive effect on female fertility.

Unexplained female infertility

Approximately 10% to 25% of infertile couples have been documented
to have unexplained infertility (Hull *et al.*, 1985; Pepperell & McBain,
1986; Templeton & Penney, 1982). The poor fertility of women with this
infertility diagnosis has been well documented. Lenton *et al.* (1977)
reported a cumulative conception rate of only 36% after seven years in
those couples with primary unexplained infertility. Templeton and Penney (1982) quoted a cumulative conception rate of 66% and 79% after 9
years of primary and secondary infertility. *In vitro* fertilization studies
have shown that oocytes obtained from women with unexplained infertility have poor fertilization rates when compared to those with tubal
disease. Therefore, it is surprising that there have been only two studies
which have suggested that unexplained infertility factors affect female
fertility and contribute substantially to failed donor insemination. This
may be because in order to make a diagnosis of unexplained female
infertility adequate screening for the presence or absence of infertility
factors must be performed prior to the commencement of inseminations.
Foss and Hull (1986) assessed conception rates in females with no
infertility factors (such as endometriosis, tubal disease and ovulatory
disorders) whose partners were azoospermic or subfertile. They found
that in those insemination recipients with azoospermic partners the
fecundability and cumulative conception rates after 12 cycles were 0.13
and 82.2% respectively. This was significantly higher ($P < 0.01$) than
those insemination recipients with subfertile partners (fecundability of
0.09 and cumulative conception rate of 66.6%). Chauhan *et al.* (1989)
have also shown that those DI recipients with no infertility factors and
azoospermic partners had significantly higher fecundability (0.18) than
those DI recipients with no infertility factors and subfertile partners, i.e.
unexplained ($P < 0.04$). This latter study also showed that the conception
rates in those with infertility factors was significantly higher than those
without factors and subfertile partners.

Age

It is widely believed that the fertility of women in the general population
decreases with increasing age. The evidence for this comes from 'natural
fertility' studies from communities which do not employ any form of
artificial methods to control fertility. One such community is the Hutterite. Tietze *et al.* (1950) showed that fertile Hutterite women had a child

for every two years of marriage and the mean age of last confinement was 40.9 years. It has been estimated for this community that the peak of fertility was at the age of 22, when seven out of every ten women had a live birth, the fertility of these women then gradually declined so that at 29 and 46 years of age, one in three and one in nine Hutterite women had a child (Tietze *et al.*, 1950; Tietze, 1957). Other 'natural fertility' studies (Henry, 1961) have reported a similar decline in fertility with increasing age.

In order to assess the true effect of age on female fertility, it is important to consider the effects of other variables which may also be detrimental to female fertility. These variables include increasing age of the partner, reduced coital frequency, increasing duration of marriage, effects of sexually transmitted disease and voluntary control of fertility. Semen collected from men of proved fertility undergoing vasectomy or screening as potential semen donors has shown significant decline in sperm motility and morphological characteristics (Schwartz *et al.*, 1983) with increasing age. Tietze (1956) showed that as coital frequency increases the percentage of women conceiving also increases. These authors noted that at a mean frequency of intercourse of once per week, the percentage conceiving in 6 months was 16.7 while in those having coitus four times per week the percentage conceiving in 6 months was 83.3%. Page (1977) and Mineau and Trussell (1982) estimated the fertility of a group of Mormon women in which the effects of decreasing fertility with increasing age of the spouse, increasing duration of marriage (decreased sexual activity) and the possible impairment of fertility with the complications of childbirth (such as puerperal infection) were also considered. The results showed little change in fertility until after 40 years of age. Menken, Trussel and Larken (1986) estimated the decline in fertility with ageing in seven groups of women in whom the decline in fertility was attributed to the result of complications of childbirth, e.g. puerperal infection. These authors concluded that the risk of childless-ness rose from 6% for 20–24 year olds, to 9% for those 25–29 year olds and to 15% for those over the age of 30 at marriage. The use of voluntary control of fertility such as the oral contraceptive pill and intrauterine contraceptive device may lead to increased sexual promiscuity with increased risk of pelvic infection (Jones *et al.*, 1982; Curran, 1980) and hence tubal disease and tubal blockage (West *et al.*, 1982; Hull *et al.*, 1985). This may be a complicating factor in estimating the true effect of age on natural fertility. However, it has been suggested that these factors are not common causes of infertility (West *et al.*, 1982; Hull *et al.*, 1985) and therefore the observed effect of age is unlikely to be due to these factors.

Therefore, there is a lot of evidence to suggest that in the general community, increasing female age is associated with decreasing fertility. However, in the general infertile population the effect of age is controversial. Collins *et al*. (1983) assessed the factors that determine treatment independent pregnancy rates in 1145 infertile couples. This study showed that the age of the wife was not a significant variable. Similarly Sorenson (1980) assessed the relative importance of various female infertility factors in determining the outcome of 196 infertile couples. Age was not a significant factor in determining the outcome. Hull *et al*. (1985) assessed the importance of age in infertile women with no infertility factors (such as tubal disease, ovulatory disorders, pelvic adhesions) and reported a significant ($P > 0.05$) decline in conception rates only after 35 years of age.

The effect of age on female fertility in a donor insemination population is also controversial. Some studies have suggested that fertility decreases with increasing age (Schwartz, 1982; Kovacs *et al*., 1988; Virro & Shewchuk 1987) and some that have suggested that there is no effect (Corson 1980; Mahadevan *et al*., 1982; Katzorke *et al*., 1981; Albrecht *et al*., 1983). Some early studies reported that age had no effect on the pregnancy rates of donor insemination recipients. Corson (1980) showed that there was no significant difference in the mean age of those that conceived (28 years) and those that failed to conceive (29 years). Similarly Katzorke *et al*. (1981) also noticed no variation in fertility with changes in age. Mahadevan *et al*. (1982) showed decreasing pregnancy rates with increasing age but this was not significant. Meeks *et al* (1986) noted from a series of 90 donor insemination recipients that those under 30 years of age had a pregnancy rate of 54% which was not significantly different from those over 30 years of age (pregnancy rate of 58%). However, the statistical analysis of the results on which these conclusions were based did not utilize life table analysis to assess conception rates and did not study the effects of age in variously subdivided age ranges. More recently, Bradshaw *et al*. (1987) found no significant difference in the cumulative conception rates of those DI recipients over 30 years of age when compared to those under 30 years. It was surprising that, in this study which primarily compared conception rates in those with ovulatory disorders and tubal disease to those without these factors, the DI recipients with these factors were not excluded from the analysis when assessing the effects of age.

In 1982 Schwartz and Mayaux assessed fecundity of 2193 partners of azoospermic men. This study reported data from 11 insemination centres using cryopreserved semen. The data were reported using life table analysis. They showed that female fertility dropped significantly after the age of 30 ($P < 0.03$) and was even more significant after 35 years of age ($P < 0.001$) when compared to those under 30 years of age. A study by Kovacs *et al.* (1988) assessed conception rates in 783 DI recipients subdivided into four age groups between 20 and 40 years of age. These authors showed that DI recipients over the age of 30 had significantly lower fertility ($P < 0.05$) than those under this age. Yeh and Seibel (1987) noted a significant ($P < 0.01$) decline in fertility after 35 years of age in 108 DI couples. Similar results have also been reported by Bergquist *et al.* (1982).

However, one major flaw in all these studies was that insemination recipients were inadequately screened for infertility factors (such as tubal disease, ovulatory disorders, pelvic adhesions and endometriosis) and those that were detected with these factors were not excluded from the analysis of the results. Therefore it is possible that this observed decline in fertility with increasing age may, in part, be due to the presence of other contributory factors such as undiagnosed infertility factors. Recently we have assessed the effect of age on the fertility of donor insemination recipients, taking into account the effect of infertility factors on female fertility. In this study, four groups of couples were studied. (1) The fertility of women with no infertility factors and azoospermic partners was studied to assess the effect of increasing age on the fertility of DI recipients *independent* of the influence of infertility factors and the semen abnormality of the partner. (2) and (3) Donor insemination recipients with infertility factors whose partners were azoospermic or subfertile respectively were studied to assess the interaction of age and infertility factors on the infertility of these recipients. (4) Donor insemination recipients with no infertility factors and subfertile partners were studied to assess the interaction of age with the semen abnormality of the partner independent of female infertility factors (Chauhan & Barratt, unpublished data).

The results of this study showed that the effect of age was different in each of the four groups of donor insemination recipients studied. In DI recipients with no infertility factors and azoospermic partners there was a significant ($P < 0.05$) decline in female fertility with increasing age. There was also a significant ($P < 0.01$) decline in the fertility of donor insemination recipients with infertility factors and subfertile partners.

However, there was no decline in the fertility of insemination recipients with infertility factors and azoospermic partners and insemination recipients with no infertility factors and subfertile partners with increasing age.This study clearly illustrated that although the effect of increasing age is to decrease female fertility, this age effect interacts with the presence of infertility factors and the semen abnormality of the partner to determine the potential fertility of donor insemination recipients.

Prognostic guidelines for DI couples

On the basis of the above discussion clinicians practising donor insemination should aim to provide prognostic guidelines to all potential couples as to the likely outcome of donor insemination. Potential DI couples can be divided into four prognostically different groups.

(a) Azoospermic partners / females with no infertility factors
(b) Azoospermic partners / females with infertility factors
(c) Subfertile partners / females with no infertility factors
(d) Subfertile partners / females with infertility factors

The probability of conception in each of these groups is different. At present there has been only one study in the literature which has assessed the conception rates in relation to these groups (Chauchan *et al.*, 1989). This study showed that DI recipients with no infertility factors whose partners were azoospermic (group (a)) had the highest fecundability (0.18) whereas those with no infertility factors whose partners were subfertile (group (c)) had the lowest fecundability (0.036). Donor insemination recipients with infertility factors (such as endometriosis, ovulatory disorders, pelvic adhesions and fibroids) whose partners were azoospermic or subfertile (groups (b) and (d)) had similar fecundability (0.05 and 0.06). The cumulative conception graphs of these four groups are illustrated in Fig. 9.1. The above groups can be used to provide prognostic guidelines as to the outcome of donor insemination and to enable clinicians to identify females with varying fertility.

The above prognostic guidelines can be used as a baseline for future development. They should be expanded by further defining the influence of individual fertility factors and their various combinations on female fertility.

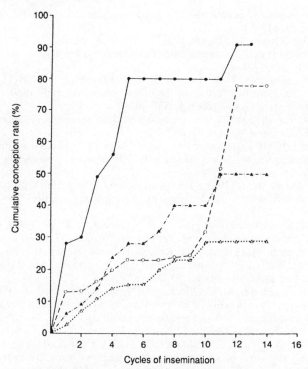

Fig. 9.1 Cumulative conception rates of donor insemination recipients. ● — ●, Azoospermic men. Females with no infertility factors. ○ – – ○, Azoospermic men. Females with infertility factors. ▲ –·–· ▲, Subfertile men. Females with infertility factors. △ · · · △, Subfertile men. Females with no infertility factors.

References

Albrecht, B. H., Cramer, D. & Schiff, I. (1982). Factors influencing the success of artificial insemination. *Fertility and Sterility*, **37**, 792–7.

Barratt, C. L. R., Chauhan, M., Cooke, I. D. (1990). Donor insemination – a look to the future. *Fertility and Sterility*, **54**, 375–87.

Bergquist, C. A., Rock, J. A., Miller, J., Guzick, D. S., Wentz, A. C. & Jones, G. S. (1982). Artificial insemination with fresh donor semen using the cervical cap technique: a review of 278 cases. *Obstetrics and Gynaecology*, **60**, 195–9.

Bordson, B. L., Ricci, E., Dickey, R. P., Dunaway, H., Taylor, S. N. & Curole, D. N. (1986). Comparison of fecundability with fresh and frozen semen in therapeutic donor insemination. *Fertility and Sterility*, **46**, 466–9.

Bradshaw, K. D., Guzick, D. S., Gruin, B., Johnson, N. & Ackerman, G. (1987). Cumulative pregnancy rates for donor insemination according to ovulatory function and tubal status. *Fertility and Sterility*, **48**, 1051–4.

Chauhan, M. C., Barratt, C. L. R., Cooke, S. & Cooke, I. D. (1989). Differences in the fertility of donor insemination recipients – a study to provide prognostic guidelines as to success and outcome. *Fertility and Sterility*, **51**, 815–19.

Collins, J. A., Wrixon, W., James, L. B. & Wilson, E. H. (1983). Treatment-independent pregnancy among infertile couples. *New England Journal of Medicine*, **309**, 1201–6.

Cooke, I. D., Sulaiman, R. A., Lenton, E. A. & Parsons, R. J. (1981). Fertility and infertility statistics : their importance and applications. *Clinics in Obstetrics and Gynaecology*, **8**, 531–48.

Corson, S. L. (1980). Factors affecting donor artificial insemination success rates. *Fertility and Sterility*, **33**, 415–22.

Curran, J. W. (1980). Economic consequences of pelvic inflammatory disease in the United States. *American Journal of Obstetrics and Gynaecology*, **138**, 848–51.

Eaton, J. & Mayer, A. J. (1953). The social biology of very high fertility among the Hutterites, the demography of a unique population. *Human Biology*, **25**, 206–64.

Emperaire, J. C., Gauzere-Soumireu, E. & Audebert, A. J. M. (1982). Female fertility and donor insemination. *Fertility and Sterility*, **37**, 90–3.

Foss, G. L. & Hull, M. G. R. (1986). Results of donor insemination related to specific male infertility and unsuspected female infertility. *British Journal of Obstetrics and Gynaecology*, **93**, 275–8.

Gillett, W. R., Camerou, M. C., MacKay-Duff, M. & Seddon, R. J. (1986). Pregnancy rates with artificial insemination by donor: the influence of the cryopreservation method and co-existent infertility factors. *New Zealand Medical Journal*, **99**, 892–3.

Hammond, M. G., Jordan, S. & Sloan, C. S. (1986). Factors affecting pregnancy rates in a donor insemination programme using frozen semen. *American Journal of Obstetrics and Gynaecology*, **155**, 480–5.

Hargreave, T. B. & Elton, R. A. (1985). Fecundability rates from an infertile male population. *British Journal of Urology*, **58**, 194–7.

Henry, L. (1961). Some data on natural fertility. *Eugenics Quarterly*, **8**, 81–91.

Hull, M. G. R., Glazener, C. M. A., Kelly, N. J., Conway, D. I., Foster, P. A., Hinton, R. A., Couldon, C., Lambert, P. A., Watt, E. M. & Desai, K. M. (1985). Population study of causes, treatment and outcome of infertility. *British Medical Journal*, **291**, 1693–7.

Jansen, R. P. S. (1986). Minimal endometriosis and reduced fecundability: prospective evidence from an artificial insemination by donor program. *Fertility and Sterility*, **46**, 141–3.

Jones, R. B., Ardery, B. R., Hui, S. L. & Cleary, R. E. (1982). Correlation between serum antichlamydial antibodies and tubal factor as a cause of infertility. *Fertility and Sterility*, **38**, 553–8.

Katayama, K. P., Kap-Soon, J. U., Manuel, M., Jones, G. S. & Jones, H. (1979). Computer analysis of etiology and pregnancy rate in 636 cases of primary infertility. *American Journal of Obstetrics and Gynaecology*, **135**, 207–14.

Katzorke, T., Propping, D. & Tauber, P. F. (1981). Results of donor artificial insemination (AID) in 415 couples. *International Journal of Fertility*, **26**, 260–6.

Kovacs, G. F., Baker, G., Burger, H., de Kretzer, D., Lording, D. & Lee, J. (1988). Artificial insemination with cryopreserved donor semen: a decade of experience. *British Journal of Obstetrics and Gynaecology*, **95**, 354–60.

Kremer, J. (1982). Voetangels en Klemmen bij donorinseminatie. *Ned Tijdschr Geneeskd.* **126**, 889–92.

Lenton, E. A., Weston, G. A. & Cooke, I. D. (1977). Long term follow-up of the apparently normal couple with a complaint of infertility. *Fertility and Sterility*, **28**, 913–19.

Mahadevan, M. M., Trounson, A. O., Milne, B. J. & Leeton, J. F. (1982). Effects of factors related to the recipients and insemination characteristics on the success of artificial insemination with frozen semen. *Clinical Reproduction and Fertility*, **1**, 195–204.

Mayaux, M. J., Schwartz, D., Czyglik, F. & David, G. (1985). Conception rate according to semen characteristics in a series of 15 364 insemination cycles: results of a multivariate analysis. *Andrologia*, **17**, 9–15.

Meeks, R. H., Judij, M., Gookin, K. M. S. N. & Bates W. G. (1986). Insemination with fresh donor semen. *Obstetrics and Gynaecology*, **68**, 527–30.

Menken, J., Trussell, J. & Larken, U. (1986). Age and fertility. *Science*, **233**: 1389–94.

Mineau, G. P. & Trussell, J. (1982). A specification of marital fertility by parents' age, age at marriage and marital duration. *Demography*, **19**, 335–49.

Page, H. J. (1977). Patterns underlying fertility schedules : a decomposition by both age and marriage duration. *Population Studies*, **31**, 85–106.

Pepperell, R. J. & McBain, J. C. (1985). Unexplained infertility : a review. *British Journal of Obstetrics and Gynaecology*, **91**, 569–80.

Schwartz, D. & Mayaux, M. J. (1982). Female fecundity as a function of age. *New England Journal of Medicine*, 404–6.

Schwartz, D., Mayaux, M. J., Spira, A., Moscato, M-L., Jouannet, P. & Czylik, F. (1983). Semen characteristics as a function of age in 833 fertile men. *Fertility and Sterility*, **39**, 530–5.

Seibel, M. M., Berger, M. J., Weinstein, F. G. & Taymor, M. L. I. (1982). The effectiveness of danazol on subsequent fertility in minimal endometriosis. *Fertility and Sterility*, **38**, 534–7.

Smith, K. D., Rodriquez-Rigau, L. J. & Steinberger, E. (1981). The influence of ovulatory dysfunction and timing of insemination on the success of artificial insemination donor (AID) with fresh or cryopreserved semen. *Fertility and Sterility*, **36**, 496–502.

Sorenson, S. S. (1980). Infertility factors: their relative importance and share in an unselected material of infertility patients. *Acta Obstetrica Gynaecologia Scandinavia*, **59**, 513–20.

Strathy, J. H., Molgaard, C. A., Coulam, C. B. & Melton, L. J. (1982). Endometriosis and infertility: a laparoscopic study of endometriosis among fertile and infertile women. *Fertility and Sterility*, **38**, 667–72.

Templeton, A. A. & Penney, G. C. (1982). The incidence, characteristics and prognosis of patients whose infertility is unexplained. *Fertility and Sterility*, **37**, 175–82.

Thomas, E. J. & Cooke, I. D. (1987). Successful treatment of asymptomatic endometriosis: does it benefit infertile women? *British Medical Journal*, **294**, 1117–19.

Tietze, C., Guttmacher, A. F. & Rubin, S. (1950). Time required for conception in 1721 planned pregnancies. *Fertility and Sterility*, **1**, 338–46.

Tietze, C. (1956). Statistical contributions to the study of human fertility. *Fertility and Sterility*, **7**, 88–95.

Tietze, C. (1957). Reproductive span and rate of reproduction among Hutterite women. *Fertility and Sterility*, **8**, 89–97.

Vessey, M. P., Wright, N. H., McPherson, K. & Wiggins, P. (1978). Fertility after stopping different methods of contraception. *British Medical Journal*, **1**, 265–7.

Virro, M. R. & Shewchuk, A. B. (1987). Pregnancy outcome in 242 conceptions after artificial insemination with donor sperm and effects of maternal age on the prognosis for successful pregnancy. *American Journal of Obstetrics*.

West, C. P., Templeton, A. A. & Lees, M. M. (1982). The diagnostic classification and prognosis of 400 infertile couples. *Infertility*, **5**, 127–44.

Westoff, C. F., Potter, R. G., Sagi, P. C. & Mishler, E. G. (1961). *Family Growth in Metropolitan America*. Princeton: Princeton University Press.

Whitelaw, M. J., Kalman, C. F. & Grams, L. R. (1970). The significance of the high ovulation rate versus the low pregnancy rate with clomid. *American Journal of Obstetrics and Gynaecology*, **107**, 865–9.

Williams, T. J. & Pratt, J. H. (1977). Endometriosis in 1000 consecutive celiotomies: incidence and management. *American Journal of Obstetrics and Gynaecology*, **129**, 245–50.

Yeh, J. & Seibel, M. M. (1987). AI with donor sperm: a review of 108 patients. *Obstetrics and Gynaecology, New York*, **70**, 313–16.

10

American organization of sperm banks

G. M. CENTOLA

Introduction

It has been over 35 years since Bunge and Sherman demonstrated that human semen could be frozen, thawed and inseminated, with a resultant normal child (Bunge & Sherman, 1953). Sherman (1965) first suggested the use of sperm banks as repositories for human semen. Although the science of cryopreservation has slowly progressed since these early developments, the organization of sperm banking facilities has changed quite dramatically since the 1950s.

Sperm banking facilities were primarily housed in universities in the 1950s and 1960s. With greater public understanding and acceptance of the procedure of sperm banking, and along with it, artificial insemination (DI) by donor DI, private banks were established in the 1970s to meet the need to freeze homologous semen prior to vasectomy, or cancer treatments, and heterologous donor semen (Sherman, 1975, 1976). By 1973, 564 normal children had been born as a result of DI with frozen semen (Sherman, 1973). In a 1986 survey of hospital-based sperm banks in the US, approximately 35 public facilities had been in existence for an average of 8.5 years, and 32 private facilities had been in operation for an average of 10 years (W. Schlaff, personal communication). Approximately 11 major commercial sperm banks and well over 50 hospital-based facilities were identified in the mid-1980s in the United States (OTA, 1988; Centola, 1989). Furthermore, it is difficult to estimate the number of small facilities in individual physician's offices and academic medical centres, since all are not registered with organizations such as the American Association of Tissue Banks (AATB) or American Fertility Society (AFS). Most major medical centre infertility units providing andrology-male infertility programmes also provide insemination with donor semen. Sperm banks for DI are often available in these units as well. A recent survey of laboratory procedures for cryopreservation of semen identified 135 facilities in the United States, although only 70 responded to the survey (Critser & Ruffing, personal communication). Increased regulations, stricter controls and increased liability, as well as the necessity for more rigorous donor screening, has resulted in the closing of many private and university-based facilities.

The 1980s have seen renewed interest in the use of frozen donor semen for DI. The demand for donor semen has been directed by an increased awareness of male infertility, and by the predominant use of 'irreversible' vasectomy as a means of contraception in the 1970s (Centola, 1989). The risks of disease transmission, particularly acquired immune deficiency syndrome (AIDS) has also shifted the demand for use of frozen donor semen (Peterson, Alexander & Moghissi, 1988).

Government intervention

In August 1988, the Office of Technology Assessment (OTA) United States Congress released results of a survey of physician and sperm bank practice in the US (OTA, 1988). During the period of June to August, 1987, two physician populations – a cross-sectional sample of primary care and reproductive care specialities, and a national probability sample of Fertility Society members – were surveyed by mail.

This survey pointed out that 172 000 women underwent DI in 1986–87 (OTA, 1988). This resulted in 35 000 births from DI with husband semen, and 30 000 births from DI. The average cost per patient for DI was $953 (US dollars) for a total of well over 150 million dollars to obtain this service from almost 11 000 physicians nationwide. Physicians reported that 51% of the women had insurance coverage for approximately 48% of the total cost. Thus, recipients were paying three-quarters of the costs themselves.

The OTA report confirmed certain findings, first reported in 1979, concerning donor screening practices. In 1979, physicians generally selected the donors themselves presumably from residents, students and other physicians, rather than purchase sperm from a commercial facility, which provided only 52% of physicians with specimens (Curie-Cohen, Luttrell & Shapiro, 1979). At the time of the OTA report, nearly one-third of physicians performing DI used fresh semen exclusively. Approximately 25% used only frozen semen, and 40% used both fresh and frozen semen.

Table 10.1. *Diagnostic testing of semen donors 1987*

	Physicians	Sperm banks
HIV testing	Yes	Yes
Syphilis serology	Yes*	Yes
Gonorrhoea culture (urethral or semen)	Yes*	Yes
Serum hepatitis	Yes*	Yes
Chlamydia Trachomatis (urethral)	Yes*	Yes
Cytomegalovirus serology	Yes*	Yes*
Herpes (urethral or semen)	Yes*	Yes*

* Indicates less than 50% of those responding to the survey conducted these tests in 1986–87.
Source: Office of Technology Assessment, 1988.

According to the OTA report, genetic screening of the donors consisted of family histories taken at the time of the interview. Less than one-third of physicians performed any biochemical tests on the donors. Approximately half of the physicians performing DI required prescreening for genetic defects or diseases (OTA, 1988). A history of serious genetic disorders was the condition for the greatest proportion of donor rejection by the physicians (see Barratt, Chauhan & Cooke, 1990).

Of the sperm banking facilities surveyed by the OTA, all facilities reported a requirement for some form of genetic screening, although screening tests varied. Sperm banks were more reluctant than office-based facilities to accept donors with a family history of genetic disorders, even those that are correctable or socially tolerable. Donors would often be rejected with family histories of conditions such as haemophilia despite the fact that they could not pass on these diseases (see Chapter 2). There was, however, uniform rejection of donors with family histories of cystic fibrosis or Huntington's chorea. Thirteen of 15 sperm banks screened for genetic diseases of ethnic origin such as Tay-Sach's disease, sickle cell anaemia or thalassaemia.

According to the OTA report (OTA, 1988), all sperm banking facilities required some form of donor screening for sexually transmitted diseases, although the nature and extent of the testing varied. Table 10.1 compared the regimen of donor screening by the surveyed facilities and private practitioners. The OTA report indicated that all sperm banks screened the donors for AIDS (HIV antibody testing). The majority of sperm banks quarantined the specimens pending further testing which occurred on an average every 1.9 months, with a 1.6 month range. Hospital-based practitioners were more likely than office-based physicians to require diagnostic testing in 1986–87 (OTA, 1988). Physicians most commonly tested for infectious diseases such as those indicated (Table 10.1). In most cases, less than 50% of physicians performing the inseminations did not require screening for sexually transmitted diseases.

Furthermore, 13 of 15 sperm banks quarantined semen in 1986–87 with donor retesting on an average every 1.9 months with a 1–6 month range. In 1988, the American Association of Tissue Banks standards for sperm banking required a minimum 3-month quarantine of donor semen (AATB, 1988). Quarantine periods for physicians and sperm banks averaged 3.6 months, although one-fourth of physicians surveyed reported a 6-month quarantine period (OTA, 1988).

It is interesting to point out that the American Fertility Society (AFS) published guidelines for the use of donor semen – either fresh or frozen – as early as 1986 (AFS 1986). The AFS guidelines recommended testing for sexually transmitted diseases including AIDS. Donor screening was to be repeated at 6 month intervals. It appeared that there was relatively little impact of these guidelines on the majority of the individual practitioner's office-based facilities in 1986, with the major impact at that time on established sperm banking facilities, as indicated by the 1986–87 survey of the OTA (OTA, 1988). Donor screening for sexually transmitted infections and genetic disorders remained variable despite the AFS guidelines (Barratt, Chauhan & Cooke, 1990).

With the release of the OTA report, Senator Albert Gore recommended that the FDA should act immediately to insure the safety of artificial insemination, to establish a national data bank to store medical and genetic histories of anonymous donors, and should assist medical professionals to develop a system of quality standards (OTA, 1988). Currently the FDA is initiating establishment proceedings to register and certify sperm banking facilities; the FDA is working closely with the medical community to establish these guidelines. Final provision for certification is expected within 2–3 years. The FDA policy is directed at commercial, private and hospital/university based sperm banks. There will probably be little impact on the private practitioner who has a small office-based sperm banking facility.

Semen from donors subsequently found to have been infected with the HIV virus had been used for artificial insemination in the United States, although there had been no confirmed reports of women infected from DI according to the OTA report (OTA, 1988). In Australia, four of eight recipients of frozen semen from a symptomless HIV positive donor were found to have developed HIV antibodies (Stewart *et al.*, 1985). As a result of the increased risks of AIDS transmission, as well as other sexually transmitted infections, there was a nationwide shift to the use of appropriately quarantined frozen semen from screened donors. In February 1988, the American Fertility Society (1988) as well as the Centre for Disease Control and the Food and Drug Administration (CDC, 1988), recommended that all semen used for DI be frozen and quarantined a minimum of 6 months. The AATB standards recommended a 3-month quarantine (AATB, 1988).

This policy was changed to a 6-month quarantine, effective from September 1989 (AATB, 1989). At that time, medical centre-based sperm banks and commercial facilities shifted to providing only 6 month quarantined semen, if these facilities had not already complied with the American Fertility Society and Centre for Disease Control guidelines (AFS, 1988; CDC, 1988).

Private practitioners are not named in these guidelines, and some have continued to use fresh donor semen. Furthermore, since the FDA has never regulated the practice of medicine by physicians, the FDA regulations will have little impact on those private practitioners with office-based sperm banks, or those who continue to provide fresh donor semen in the office setting. In these instances, donor screening is often quite variable, minimal or non-existent.

New York State (NYS) is one of only four states with specific regulations for sperm banks (NYS, 1989). The four states in addition to New York are Illinois, Indiana and Michigan. A total of 12 states have laws requiring HIV antibody testing of semen donors. The NYS regulations became effective October 1989. These regulations call for the sole use of 6-month quarantined frozen donor semen for DI (NYS, 1989). Donor and recipient confidentiality is guaranteed by the regulations. Records must be maintained for 22 years.

Additionally, the NYS regulations indicate that sperm banking facilities operating in the state, or shipping into the state, must be approved and certified by the NYS Department of Health. The procedure for certification includes submission of a protocol and operations policy to the state officials, and yearly on-site inspection. The mandated donor screening regimen is shown in Table 10.2. Screening for AIDS must be accomplished initially, after a minimum 6-month quarantine, and prior to release of the semen for artificial insemination.

Table 10.2. *Semen donor screening protocol*

Initial[a]	Six month
Hepatitis B Surface Ag	*HIV/HTLV-1 exposure
Hepatitis B Core Ab	Hepatitis C
Hepatitis C	All others at six month intervals
Alanine aminotransferase	
HIV/HTLV-1	
Chlamydia trachomatis (urethral or semen swab)	
Neisseria gonorrhoea (urethral or semen swab)	
Cytomegalovirus	
Rh/ABO Blood type	

Semen quality (motility, density) of each specimen must be assessed using standard, accepted procedures.

[a] Tests on serum unless otherwise indicated.
* Prior to release of the donor semen after six month quarantine, the donor must be tested for HIV/HTLV-1 exposure.
Source: New York State Department of Health, 1989, 1992.

These NYS regulations have had a major impact on sperm banking and artificial insemination practice in New York State. Although the regulations are aimed at protecting the patient from disease transmission, and the facility and physician from liability, the increased screening regimen has led to increased costs. At a time when medical costs are under close scrutiny by government officials and medical insurance carriers, the increased costs of DI are sure to come under fire by consumer advocates and government officials. Unfortunately, not all facilities and private practitioners are in compliance with these state regulations. It is difficult and perhaps impossible to monitor artificial insemination practice. Sperm banking facilities are perhaps the easiest to regulate within the constraints of law. Regulation of sperm banks has, without a doubt, impacted on the practice of DI in NYS, and will continue to affect this aspect of infertility treatment well into the future.

Impact of AIDS

Over the past several years, the increased risk of AIDS in the heterosexual population has had tremendous impact on sperm banking practice in the US. The American Fertility Society revised its 1986 guidelines for donor semen in 1988 and again in 1990 as a result of these apparent risks (AFS, 1986, 1988, 1990). Sexual transmission of the HIV virus is the most common mechanism of transmission, yet it is the most poorly understood (Alexander, 1990). Furthermore, the virus, although lethal, is poorly transmitted (May, Anderson & Blower, 1989; Alexander, 1990). Many sexually transmitted infections are more efficiently transmitted than HIV (Alexander, 1990). Compounding this, is the fact that the mean incubation period from **seroconversion to AIDS** is 8 to 10 years (Bacchetti & Moss, 1989; Alexander, 1990). Current standards (NYS, 1989; AATB, 1990) set quarantine time for frozen donor semen at a minimum of 6 months. Of additional impact on sperm banking facilities has been a recommendation of hepatitis C (HCV) testing of semen donors (Sherman, personal communication). Prequarantine HCV testing of semen donors is not available since serum samples are generally not stored long-term on all donors. This may have disastrous effect on several sperm banking facilities (Sherman, personal communication). Since October, 1989, the NYS Department of Health has recommended alanine aminotransferase screening (liver enzyme) for non-A and non-B forms of hepatitis, which substituted for the HCV test until it recently became available. However, revised NYS regulations will call for actual HCV testing in addition to all other tests currently performed for hepatitis screening (NYS Department of Health, 1991, 1992). The Reproductive Council of AATB is suggesting that all sperm banking facilities keep serum samples of all donors stored for future testing as improved methods of detection become available (Sherman, personal communication).

The major effect of AIDS, and thus of using only frozen donor semen for DI generally revolves around the costs and effectiveness of the frozen semen (Peterson *et al.*, 1988). Management of sperm banking facilities with emphasis on quality assurance and quality control measures has been improved as a result of the AIDS crisis and sperm banking regulations. With the implementation of HIV/HTLV-1 testing of semen donors (NYS, 1989) and the extended quarantine since 1988, questions arise as to the impact on semen stored prior to 1988. This is similar to the concerns raised by the recommendations for HCV testing of donors.

The risk of disease transmission, the sole use of frozen semen for DI and national and state regulations have had a major impact on the infrastructure of sperm banks. Small facilities with a small donor pool and small recipient population appear to be easiest to manage. However, logistic management of donor screening protocols as well as specimen handling for DI have become favourable tasks for larger facilities, particularly the commercial banks. Some facilities suggest maintenance of a long-term relationship with semen donors for routine screening, particularly after a donor has stopped participating in the programme. One commercial facility maintains contact for five years (Anouna, personal communication).

Sperm banking in the 1990s

Government involvement, both on a state and federal level, has already had a major impact on sperm banking in the United States. With increasing government involvement in sperm banking specifically, and donor insemination in general, it is anticipated that smaller facilities, and practitioner based sperm banks will be forced to close their programmes. Smaller facilities incapable of meeting the guidelines or state standards will not survive in this arena. Facilities may also close rather than accept the increased liability related to providing this service. Larger facilities, particularly commercial, for-profit facilities are capable of bearing the increased costs of licensing/certification. Increased research will improve outcome of DI with frozen semen (see Chapter 6). Ultimately, however, the increased cost will be passed on to the patient and the medical insurance companies. The costs of these services are already overwhelming (OTA, 1988). In the future, the medical insurance companies will undoubtedly be forced to cover a portion of these expenses.

Throughout this decade, the clinicians, scientists, politicians and lay persons together can foster an atmosphere of cooperation aimed at providing safe DI care. Ultimately, the establishment of national standards for certification of sperm banking facilities will insure a safe product for the patient. The American Association of Tissue Banks and The American Fertility Society have been in the vanguard in this respect, working closely with the government and scientific community to insure not only safe DI, but also to assess scientific and medical practicability and accuracy of proposed standards. These national and state regulations are aimed at reducing the liability to the facility and the physician at a time when the medical–legal climate is threatening. The future can be looked to with guarded, cautious optimism.

References

Alexander, N. J. (1990). Sexual transmission of human immunodeficiency virus: entry into the male and female genital tract. *Fertility and Sterility*, **54**, 1–18.

American Association of Tissue Banks (1988). *Standards for Tissue Banking.* Arlington, Virginia: AATB.
American Association of Tissue Banks (1989). *Standards for Tissue Banking.* Arlington, Virginia: AATB.
American Fertility Society (1986). New guidelines for the use of semen donor insemination: 1986. *Fertility and Sterility*, **46**(Suppl. 2), 95S-110S.
American Fertility Society (1988). Revised new guidelines for the use of semen donor insemination. *Fertility and Sterility*, **49**, 211–12.
American Fertility Society (1990). New guidelines for the use of semen donor insemination: 1990. *Fertility and Sterility*, **53**(Suppl 10), 1S-13S.
Bacchetti, P. & Moss, A. R. (1989). Incubation period of AIDS in San Francisco. *Nature*, **338**, 251.
Bunge, R. G. & Sherman, J. K. (1953). Fertilizing capacity of frozen human spermatozoa. *Nature*, **172**, 767.
Center for Disease Control (1988). Semen banking, organ and tissue transplantation and HIV antibody testing. *Morbidity and Mortality Weekly Report* **37**, 1.
Centola, G. M. (1989). Effect of cryopreservation on human sperm motility. *Molecular Andrology*, **1**, 399–412.
Curie-Cohen, M., Luttrell, L. & Shapiro, S. (1979). Current practice of artificial insemination by donor in the United States. *New England Journal of Medicine*, **300**, 585–90.
May, R. M., Anderson, R. M. & Blower, S. M. (1989). The epidemiology and transmission dynamics of HIV-AIDS. *Daedalus*, **118**, 163.
New York State Department of Health (1989). *Human Semen Banking.* Subpart 58-7, Part 58 of title 10 (Health) of the Official Compilation of Codes, Rules and Regulations of the State of New York. New York: Public Health Council (revised 1991, 1992).
Office of Technology Assessment (OTA), Congress of the United States (1988). *Artificial Insemination Practice in the United States. Summary of a 1987 Survey.* Background Paper. Washington, DC: Office of Technology Assessment, Congressional Board of the 100th Congress, US Congress.
Peterson, E. P., Alexander, N. J. & Moghissi, K. S. (1988). AID and AIDS – too close for comfort. *Fertility and Sterility*, **49**, 209–10.
Sherman, J. K. (1965). Practical applications and technical problems of preserving spermatozoa by freezing. *Federation Proceedings*, **24**, 288.
Sherman, J. K. (1973). Synopsis of the use of frozen human semen since 1964: State of the art of human semen banking. *Fertility and Sterility*, **24**, 397–412.
Sherman, J. K. (1975). Research on frozen human semen. *Fertility and Sterility*, **15**, 487.
Sherman, J. K. (1976). Clinical use of frozen human semen. *Transplant Proceedings*, **8**, 165a.
Stewart, G. J., Cunningham, A. L., Driscoll, G. L., Tyler, J. P. P., Barr, J. A., Gold, J., Lamont, B. J. (1985). Transmission of human T-cell lymphotropic virus type III (HTLV-III) by artificial insemination by donor. *Lancet*, **ii**, 581–5.

11

Artificial procreation with frozen donor semen: the French experience of CECOS

FEDERATION CECOS, D. LE LANNOU
and J. LANSAC

Introduction: general procedure

Artificial insemination with donor semen is an old method for treating male infertility. As in other countries, this method of treatment in France was originally performed using fresh semen with no opportunity for regulation. The establishment of sperm banks has permitted the installation of strict controls for semen donation and recipient couple selection (Steinberger & Smith, 1973; Trounson et al., 1979; David & Lansac, 1980; Albrecht, Cramer & Schiff, 1982; Bordson et al., 1986).

In 1973, the first sperm banks began operating in France, each under the auspices of a CECOS (Centre d'Etude et de Conservation du Sperme Humain). Each CECOS bank operates according to the same guidelines and management principles, in accordance with the philosophy formulated by G. David, that 'all sperm donations must be given voluntarily without payment and the donations must come from a couple who have one or more children'. There are now 20 CECOS in France united by a charter of Federation. There is an annual nationwide evaluation of their activities (Federation CECOS, Le Lannou & Lansac 1989). The general procedures for donor recruitment, semen cryopreservation and selection of recipient couples are the same in all CECOS.

Donors: recruitment and selection

All semen donors are from couples with one or more children. This donation is anonymous and non-paid, although donors can be compensated for travelling expenses.

152

Table 11.1. *Recruitment of donors in*
CECOS 1973–1988

Unsolicited volunteers	1803	(24.2%)
Referred by DI candidates	2852	(38.3%)
Vasectomy	1676	(22.5%)
Referred by gynaecologists	665	(8.9%)
Other	434	(5.8%)
	7430	

This requirement, which is specific to the CECOS, offers several advantages: there is an additional guarantee of donor fertility as well as a lower risk of hereditary disease, these men respond honestly to the personal and family medical screening and they represent a population with a very low risk of AIDS (3000 donors so far have been tested for HIV, none were positive).

Recruitment of donors

The recruitment of donors is for the CECOS, as for all sperm banks, a major problem. Since 1973, 8860 couples considered semen donation within the CECOS system. A review of this donor recruitment revealed three main groups (Table 11.1):

1. Unsolicited volunteers, being couples informed through the mass media.
2. Donors responding to pleas by DI recipient candidates. These can be relatives or close friends of the couples seeking DI treatment (the DI recipients are told that any donors recruited by them will not be used for their own treatment).
3. Vasectomy patients: in France many surgeons who perform vasectomies recommend semen cryopreservation to their patients, specifically with a view to its possible use later by the patients themselves. They are also given information about semen donation; currently one third of all vasectomy patients become semen donors.

Candidate donors return five to six times to CECOS to make semen donations.

The number of pregnancies obtained using any donor's semen is restricted in order to limit the risk of consanguinity (on average five children per donor (see Chapter 3 for the risks of consanguinity and number of acceptable pregnancies). Despite recruitment difficulties and restrictive selection criteria, can CECOS satisfy all the demand for DI treatment? When estimating the number of donors needed to meet this demand, three points must be considered (Le Lannou, Lobel & Chambon, 1980): fewer than 50% of women seeking DI achieve pregnancies in the best results so far reported, no more than five pregnancies are allowed for a given donor, and donor selection gives a donor acceptance rate of about 60%. Theoretically the number of donors required can be calculated as follows:

Number of donors = Number of DI requests

$\times$ 50% (women who will have a child)

$\times$ 1/5 (maximum pregnancies by donor)

$\times$ 60% (selection rate of donors)

= Number of DI requests ÷ 6

This formula gives the minimum number of donors required, since all variables cannot be calculated. It is not certain, for example, that a total of five pregnancies can be achieved with each donor. In 1989 therefore, 3600 requests for DI treatment called for the recruitment of a minimum of 600 donors. In fact 740 donors were enrolled.

These results show that CECOS can be considered to be well on the way to achieving their double aim. On the one hand, to meet the demand for DI and on the other hand, to foster greater public acceptance of DI by providing maximum conditions of safety and reliability.

Selection

It is generally admitted that donors must be selected (Barratt and Cooke, 1989, AFS, 1990); the aim of this selection is twofold:

1. to select fertile semen to give couples a better chance of success;
2. to prevent the transmission of serious diseases, for the recipient (infectious disease) and for the child to be born (hereditary disease).

Fertile semen

Two approaches can be used to recruit fertile men: first the recruitment of men who have fathered a child, and second, the recruitment of men with semen characteristics above minimal limits. In France, these two approaches are used simultaneously: all semen donors are from couples with one or more children and ejaculates are analysed both before and after cryopreservation. The criteria for selection are based upon the post-thaw characteristics, particularly post-thaw motility. CECOS only recommend the use of straws with >30% motility and >2 million total motile spermatozoa.

Transmission of infectious diseases

The risk of transmission of infectious diseases can be minimized by medical screening including complete sexual history, sperm cultures and blood tests (syphilis, hepatitis, HIV) (see Chapter 2).

HIV screening is now the major problem. Donors in CECOS are very low risk for HIV as they are men living in a stable relationship. The HIV serological testing is performed at the time of the last donation and the frozen semen is quarantined for six months. The donor is again tested for HIV following that period. Since 1973, 8860 couples have volunteered for semen donation. Less than 1% of the donors were excluded for risks of sexually transmitted diseases. HIV serological testing of a sub-population of 1436 women inseminated between 1981 (the beginning of the spread of AIDS in France) and 1985 (beginning of systematic serological HIV screening of semen donors in France) produced completely negative findings. Since 1985, HIV serology has been systematic for all potential donors, there have been no positive results in 3000 cases.

Transmission of hereditary diseases

Possible transmission of hereditary diseases can be minimized by karyotyping and genetic screening of potential donors (Selva *et al.*, 1986, Jalbert *et al.*, 1989). Among 676 prospective donors, 8.6% had chromosomal abnormalities, but only 3.6% of these were rejected since some of the anomalies were considered variants. The usefulness of a karyotype for all donors is evident from this study.

The risk of transmission of hereditary disease can also be minimized by genetic screening of donors through family and personal history. The results of this screening depend on: the competence level of the interviewer (physician or geneticist), the precision of the questionnaire, and the degree of expected safety. It is obvious that a threshold has to be determined, for if every carrier of recessive genes were rejected, and if all heterozygotes could be detected, there would not be any qualified donors! For these reasons, CECOS decided to classify candidate donors into three groups: 1) rejected, 2) accepted without restrictions, 3) accepted with specific risk factors. Concerning the last group, disorders of genetic origin (e.g. allergy) were detected through the genetic interview of the donor. Before using such semen, it was necessary to ensure that the genetic history of the recipient did not reveal the same disorder. Of the 676 donors in the study, 3.6% were totally rejected and 47% were accepted with a specific risk factor.

In total CECOS donor selection, criteria are extremely strict with only 62% of prospective donors being accepted. Of all donor candidates initially interviewed, 11% failed to return to make a donation, possibly because of insufficient motivation. Another 27% of candidates were rejected either for reasons of poor semen quality, either before or after freezing, or more rarely, for genetic reasons. Fewer than 1% of donors were excluded for risks of sexually transmitted diseases.

Use of fresh or frozen semen

DI treatment involves the risk of infection by sexually transmitted diseases. Although this risk is rather small (less than 1% in the author's series), it is not ethically permissible to take this risk. Consequently, only the use of cryopreserved donor semen with sufficiently strict control of sexually transmitted diseases, especially AIDS is acceptable (Ball, 1986). Sperm cultures for anaerobic and aerobic bacteria are performed on all donors. If the donor has a history of sexually transmitted disease, other tests on the semen are performed, e.g. chlamydia.

The same semen cryopreservation technique has been adopted throughout the CECOS Federation. A cryoprotectant medium containing glycerol and egg yolk is used and the semen is packaged in 0.25 ml straws (IMV L'Aigle, France). After a relatively rapid freezing process, the straws were stored in liquid nitrogen. Over the last 4 years, the overall MSRC (mean success rate per cycle) of the CECOS Federation is 8.5%. The cumulative success rate following DI with frozen semen is approximately 50% after the first six cycles. These results are similar to those reported previously (Trounson et al., 1981) and show very little difference to the cumulative success rates obtained with fresh semen inseminations (Bordson et al., 1986; Trounson et al., 1979). However, several studies have shown that fresh semen was more effective than cryopreserved semen (Chapter 6; Richter et al., 1984, Smith et al., 1981).

Table 11.2. *Indications for DI requests, Federation CECOS 1984–1987*

Azoospermia	4851	52.9%
Oligozoospermia $0-1\times10^6$/ml	1651	18.0%
Oligozoospermia $1-5\times10^6$/ml	1010	11.0%
Oligozoospermia $5-20\times10^6$/ml	850	9.3%
Astheno-teratozoospermia	645	7.0%
Genetic risks	162	1.8%
	9165	100.0%

Note: Oligozoospermia, teratozoospermia, astheno-teratozoospermia as defined by WHO (1987).

Nevertheless, even if fresh semen is more efficient, its use will be very limited as the numerous advantages of frozen semen are realized: constant availability, possibility of more complete control particularly bacteriological and virological, possibility of transport, possibility of performing several inseminations per cycle with the semen of the same donor and ability to store samples for clearance of HIV status.

DI requests and screening of women

The primary indication for DI recipients is male infertility. In addition to cases of irreversible male sterility, due to both secretory and obstructional azoospermia, which are obvious indications for DI, CECOS receives many requests in cases of 'sperm insufficiency', i.e. oligozoospermia, asthenozoospermia, teratozoospermia. Such cases are different because they involve subfertility and not sterility. They are accepted for DI only if all other treatments have failed to improve the couple's fertility.

The second indication for DI is the presence of genetic risks such as those due to a male dominant or recessive heritable disorder.

In CECOS all DI requests have been exclusively therapeutic, always for heterosexual couples and the proportions of the various indications are presented in Table 11.2.

Since 1973 CECOS has received about 35,000 DI requests. After an initial period of rapid growth, the requests have now stabilized at about 3000 new requests per year. This number represents nearly 1% of the

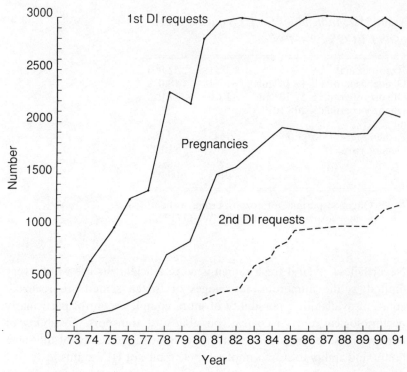

Fig. 11.1. Evolution of the DI requests and pregnancies within the CECOS Federation programme.

marriages registered yearly in France. Since 1980 there has been an appreciable increase in the number of couples who, having obtained a first child by DI, have returned to CECOS for a second or third child. These repeated DI requests now represent one-third of all requests (Fig. 11.1).

Not all of the DI recipients accepted on to the waiting lists begin inseminations. During the waiting period, which means a length of approximately 10 months, some couples drop out through insufficient motivation. Other couples with sperm insufficiency may drop out because the woman has become pregnant either spontaneously or after some form of treatment with her partner's semen. During the last 4 years, out of 15 000 requests, only 12 000 women began inseminations.

Since 1973, there have been approximately 22 000 pregnancies following DI treatment, the overall MSRC for all women who began DI was approximately 8.5%. During the last four years, 11 900 women began DI treatment and 8556 pregnancies have been obtained. The average success rate per patient was 71% including those who dropped out.

An important role of Federation CECOS has been to collate all DI results on a national level. Detailed analysis of these data has allowed DI to be used as a model for studying human fecundity, the statistical validity of this approach is enhanced by standard methods and the large number of DI cycles examined. These epidemiological studies have revealed a variety of success factors (see below).

Analysis of data

For all recipient couples an assessment of tubal patency and evidence of ovulation is required for the female partner and a semen evaluation for the husband. All couples attended an interview to discuss the psychological aspects of artificial procreation with donor semen prior to being accepted onto the waiting list. CECOS operates by distributing semen to gynaecologists either in private or hospital practice. Pregnancies are identified by positive hCG tests and all results are collected from the gynaecologists by the CECOS. The data have been evaluated using the method of life-table analysis adapted for DI (Schwartz & Mayaux, 1980). The values presented are the mean success rate per cycle (MSRC) and the theoretical cumulative success rate (TCSR) at n cycles after the exclusion of patients who had dropped out of the treatment. The efficacy of the artifical procreation with donor depends on the following factors: female fertility, semen quality, technical expertise.

Female factors

A detailed analysis of the results has shown that the women inseminated were a heterogeneous population with some of them being subfertile or infertile. This conclusion is supported by the observation that the success rate obtained for women being inseminated for a first pregnancy was lower than that obtained for women undergoing treatment for a second or third DI pregnancy (Federation CECOS & Le Lannou 1988). Clearly a higher proportion of women in the population being inseminated for a first pregnancy would be subfertile.

The MSRC was also found to be dependent upon the length of the treatment. It decreased from a mean of 10.3% over the first six cycles to 2.3% after 24 cycles of DI (Fig. 11.2).

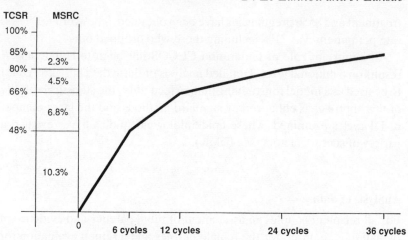

Fig. 11.2. Results of 23 700 DI cycles: theoretical cumulative success rate (TSCR) and mean success rate per cycle (MSRC) in relation to the number of cycles performed.

This decreased success rate per cycle with increasing numbers of insemination cycles can only indicate that the more fertile women conceived more readily, and therefore a greater proportion of subfertile or infertile women remained in the population still undergoing treatment with increasing numbers of cycles of inseminations. The theoretical cumulative success rate (drop-outs excluded) for all women was 48% after six cycles, 66% after 12 cycles and 80% after 24 cycles.

Studies by the CECOS Federation have revealed some female factors upon which the success rate is dependent.

Age of the women

Lower success rates have often been reported to be positively correlated with the women's age. However, this parameter is usually examined for the population of DI treated women as a whole, which may create a sampling bias. Indeed, a certain proportion of the women with non-azoospermic husbands are subfertile. This proportion increases with time: the longer the period of infertility the larger the proportion of infertile women. Therefore, a woman's age is a parameter that can truly be evaluated only in women whose husbands are azoospermic. The CECOS Federation studied 2193 women who had azoospermic husbands (Federation CECOS, Schwartz & Mayaux, 1982). It was clearly demonstrated that the DI success rate began to decrease for patients of 31 years

Table 11.3. *Results of DI according to partner's semen quality*

	Number of pregnancies	Pregnancy/cycle
Azoospermic	317	12.6%
Oligo <5 M/ml	110	12.7%
Oligo 5–20 M/ml	30	8.9%*
>20 M/ml	35	7.3%*

* $P < 0.01$.

or older, and is appreciably reduced by age 36 years when the cumulative success rate after 12 cycles of DI treatment is 54%, compared to 75% for women of less than 25 years of age.

Indication for DI

Many studies have shown that the fertility of women in the DI programme depends upon the partner's semen quality. Emperaire *et al.*, (1982) showed that out of 131 insemination recipients, the cumulative success rate was significantly higher in those patients with azoospermic partners (70%) when compared with those with subfertile partners (47%).

Another study from CECOS confirmed these results (see Table 11.3): this finding has been explained on the basis that those DI recipients married to oligozoospermic men represent a selected subfertile group from which women of normal or high fecundity have been removed by spontaneous conception.

Semen factors

Semen quality of the donor is an important source of variability in the success of DI. David *et al.* (1980), using CECOS data, showed that the most important predictor of fertilizing capacity of semen was post-thaw motility: the success rate per cycle was 7% when the post-thaw motility was <40%, and 17% when it was >65% (Table 11.4).

In another study using semen cryopreserved before chemotherapy or radiotherapy, and hence unselected for quality, it was demonstrated that no pregnancies were obtained with insemination with less than 0.5 million thawed motile spermatozoa. Using between 0.5 and 2 million motile

Table 11.4. *Success rate of DI according to donor semen characteristics (the number of cycles is given in parentheses)*

	Post-thaw motility in per cent				Number of motile spermatozoa per straw in millions		
	<40	45,50	55,60	>65	<5	5–10	>10
Cycles	7%	9%	14%	17%	7%	13%	15%
(1489)	(327)	(475)	(493)	(194)	(513)	(635)	(341)

* $P < 0.001$.

spermatozoa, the success rate was low (4% per cycle) it was 10% per cycle with insemination doses above 2 million, and it reached 15% with more than 10 million motile sperm.

A better selection of the semen that retains only semen with a post thaw motility >65%, would permit a higher success rate, but would constitute a major problem in donor recruitment, since in our donor fertile population, those semen represent only 13% of all!

Technique of insemination with donor semen

Intracervical insemination

The intracervical insemination is the most popular method. This technique is simple: after thawing, a part of the semen from the straw is inserted into the cervical mucus and the rest deposited in a cervical cap placed on the cervix.

The appropriate time for artificial insemination is usually estimated on the basis of basal body temperature charts and the examination of cervical mucus. The gynaecologist is free to decide when, and how often, inseminations should be performed and to prescribe other treatments such as induction of ovulation. Usually, one or two inseminations are performed per cycle.

Analysis of the data have shown two important factors in the practice of the DI: the timing of the insemination compared to ovulation, and the quality of cervical mucus. Studying 465 cycles with a single insemination, the date of ovulation was determined from the BBT curve and mucus cervical score analysis. An optimum period appears from day J_{-2} to day J_0 which correlates with the maximum of the cervical score (Fig. 11.3). Usually two inseminations at a 48 h interval are necessary to cover this

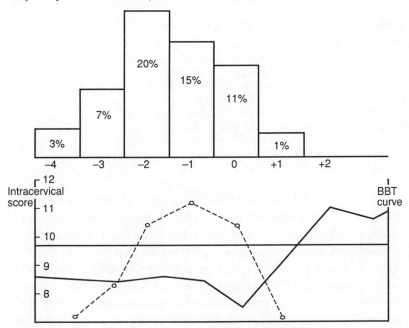

Fig. 11.3. MSRC at each day of insemination and optimum period for DI, correlated with cervical score (broken line) and BBT curve (solid line).

optimum period. The usefulness of better ovulation prediction by ultrasonography or measurement of hormone level has not been confirmed.

Other techniques

The considerable decrease in MSRC after 12 and 24 cycles of intracervical DI treatment questions the value of continuing DI for a longer period. In relation to this, the appearance of new forms of artificial procreation recently developed has caused the approach towards cases of DI failure to be reconsidered.

These new techniques are far more medically agressive but offer a better pregnancy rate.

Surgical technique such as gamete intra fallopian transfer (GIFT) or *in vitro* fertilization (IVF) have been offered to women following an unsuccessful series of intracervical DI, or sometimes at the outset when the initial gynaecological examination revealed abnormalities such as tubal occlusion (IVF). The frequency of IVFD (IVF with donor semen), GIFTD (GIFT with donor semen) relative to DI is shown in Table 11.5.

Table 11.5. *Artificial procreation with donor sperm, Federation 1988–89*

	DI	IVFD	GIFTD
Cycles	41470	3680	367
Pregnancies	3525	807	89
MSRC	8.5%	21.9%[a]	24.2%[a]

[a] Both IVFD and GIFTD are significantly ($P <$ 0.001) better than DI. $P < 0.001$.

It should be noted that the MSRC obtained by IVFD or GIFTD were considerably higher than that obtained by DI. More detailed analysis has demonstrated that the results of IVFD, like those of DI, depended upon the number of unsuccessful preceding DI cycles. Furthermore, since one woman can hope to receive a maximum of ten DI cycles or three IVFD cycles in a year, the TCSR results for these two forms of treatment can be calculated for a one year period: this demonstrates that the TCSR of ten cycles of DI or three cycles of IVFD are the same in patients who had not had any preceding DI treatment cycles. After 12 cycles of unsuccessful DI, the difference between the TCSR values for the two methods is relatively small, but becomes greater in those patients who had 24 previous cycles of unsuccessful DI treatment (Table 11.6).

Furthermore, in practice IVFD has no advantage if it is used from the outset, only becoming significantly better after approximately 18 cycles of failed DI treatment (see Chapter 8.)

Intrauterine insemination using sperm selection techniques was studied and resulted in an improved pregnancy rate compared with intracervical insemination with unprepared semen samples. In these cases, the stimulation of ovulation was systematically performed using clomiphene citrate or/and hMG with a single intrauterine insemination used 36 h after hCG. In a study from 2000 cycles of artificial procreation in one centre (Le Lannou *et al.*, 1990), the intracervical insemination DIC was used in from 1 to 12 cycles, the intrauterine insemination DIU was used in between 12 to 18 cycles and the *in vitro* fertilization IVFD after 18 cycles. The results of the different methods are noted in Table 11.7: these results showed the interest and the place of intrauterine insemination in an artificial procreation programme.

Over the last 10 years, the MSRC of intracervical insemination between 12 and 18 cycles has been approximately 5%. With intrauterine

Table 11.6. *Mean success rate per cycle (MSRC) and theoretical cumulative success rate by time (TCSR) in procreation with donor sperm*

	DI		IVFD	
	MSRC	TCSR	MSRC	TCSR
Number of previous AID cycles		10 cyc		3 cyc
0	10.3%	60.6%	26.9%[a]	60.7%
>12	4.5%	36.9%	16.8%[a]	42.3%
>24	2.3%	20.6%	16.3%[a]	41.3%[b]

[a] MSRC significantly ($P < 0.001$) between DI and IVFD.
[b] TCRS significantly ($P < 0.001$) between DI and IVFD.

Table 11.7. *Comparison between intracervical (DIC), intrauterine insemination (DIV) and in vitro fertilization (IVFD) using donor semen*

	DIC	DIU	IVFD
Cycles	1–12	12–18	>18
Success rate (MSRC)	11.0%	15.2%	16.1%
Number cycles	(1500)	(301)	(161)

Table 11.8. *Outcome of the pregnancies*

	DI	IVFD
Cycles	3246	695
Miscarriages <12 W	559 (17.2%)	168 (24.5%)
Deliveries	2575	481
Single	95.1%	72.5%
Twin	4.3%	23.0%
Triplets	0.4%	4.3%
New borns	2714	638
Sex ratio	0.98	0.98
Malformations	45 (1.6%)	4 (0.6%)

insemination, the MSRC between 12 and 18 cycles is 15%. In a random-ized study, intracervical versus intrauterine DI was compared after between 12 and 18 cycles. Intrauterine insemination was significantly better (Le Lannou *et al.*, 1989). Since then intrauterine insemination has been used systematically after 12 failed cycles.

Pregnancies

There is a paucity of studies relating to the pregnancies after DI (Lansac *et al.*, 1984); these studies are often short-term. Some authors (Forse *et al.*, 1985) have suggested an increase in the number of abnormalities in the DI offspring. Since 1987, the CECOS Federation has implemented a prospective study on pregnancies achieved by DI and their medical outcome. The first data concerning 3931 cycles with pregnancies and 3871 birth (1.5% lost to follow-up) are shown in Table 11.8.

For DI the rate of miscarriages was 17.2%. The rate of ectopic pregnancies was 1%, and 81.2% of the pregnancies were continued to delivery. Of the 2575 deliveries, 95% were single, 4% twins and 0.4% triplets or more. The sex ratio was normal, and the overall incidence of malformations, less than 2%, is lower following DI than in the general population.

The comparative results for IVFD showed a significant increase in miscarriage, and a higher rate of multiple pregnancies.

In total, it would seem that the children resulting from artificial procreation with frozen donor semen have been normal, but particularly the low incidence of chromosome abnormalities make it necessary to examine this question in a larger series.

Conclusions

In France, the CECOS is unique by virtue of its organization on a national level within the Federation. The operating principles of CECOS are very different from those practised in other countries, especially the strict controls regulating semen donation: i.e. donations are benevolent, anonymous and made by a couple. After 18 years of operation, the combined experience of the CECOS has shown that the strict application of these principles is possible on a national level.

The systemic collation and analysis of data from assisted procreation using donor semen has not only allowed improvements in selection of those patients who will be more likely to benefit from the procedure, but has also improved understanding of factors which influence natural fertility. These results have also allowed the development of better guidelines for artificial procreation by semen donor practice. Over the last five years, the overall success rate of the CECOS Federation has increased from 7.2 to 9.6%.

There are some remaining questions relating to human procreation using donor semen, notably studies on the outcome of the resulting pregnancies. Further studies are needed to consider the important psychological aspects of DI not only for the children, but also the parents and the donors (see Chapter 13.)

Acknowledgements

Federation CECOS: P. Jouannet and F. Czyglick (Paris-Bicentre), C. Da Lage and M. O. Alnot (Paris-Necker), J. P. Dadoune and J. Auger (Paris-Hotel-Dieu), F. Thepot and J. C. Boulanger (Amiens), C. Bugnon et M. C. Clavequin (Besançon), J. Meunier and J. Berjeon (Bordeaux), J. Izard and A. Sauvalle (Caen), D. Boucher and J. Janny (Clermont-Ferrand), P. Jalbert and M. Servoz-Gavin (Grenoble), M. Delecour and P. St-Pol (Lille), J. C. Czyba and D. Cottinet (Lyon), J. M. Luciani and R. Roullier (Marseille), C. Humeau and M. Chalet (Montpellier), G. Grignon and B. Foliguet (Nancy), J. J. Adnet and C. Mellin (Reims), D. Le Lannou and B. Charbonnel (Rennes), J. P. Bisson and F. Bastit (Rouen), A. Clavert (Strasbourg), F. Pontonnier and A. Mansat (Toulouse), J. Lansac and M. J. Tharanne (Tours).

References

Albrecht, B. H., Cramer, D. & Schiff, I. (1982). Factors influencing the success of artificial insemination. *Fertility and Sterility*, **37**, 792–7.

American Fertility Society (1990). Ethical considerations of the new reproductive technologies. *Fertility and Sterility*, **53**, suppl.2.

Ball, G. D. (1986). Acquired immunde deficiency syndrome and the fertility clinic. *Fertility and Sterility*, **45**, 172–4.

Barratt, C. L. R., & Cooke, I. D. (1989). Risks of donor insemination (Editorial). *British Medical Journal*, **2993**, 178.

Bordson, B. L., Ricci, E., Dickey, R. P., Dunaway, H., Taylor, S. N. & Curole, D. N. (1986). Comparison of fecundability with fresh and frozen semen in therapeutic donor insemination. *Fertility and Sterility*, **46**, 466–9.

David, G. & Lansac, J. (1980). The organisation of the centers for the study and preservation of semen in France. In *Human Artificial Insemination and Semen Preservation*. David, G. & Price, W. S. eds. pp. 15–26, New York and London: Plenum Press.

David, G., Czyglick, F., Mayaux, M. J. & Schwartz, (1980). The success of AID and semen characteristics: study on 1489 cycles and 192 ejaculates. *International Journal of Andrology*, **3**, 613–19.

Emperaire, J. C., Gauzere Soumiren, E. & Audebert, A. J. M. (1982). Female fertility and donor insemination. *Fertility and Sterility*, **37**, 90–3.

Federation CECOS & Le Lannou, D. (1988). Bilan de l'activité des CECOS. *Contraception, Fertility and Sexuality*, **16**, 547–9.

Federation CECOS, Schwartz, D. & Mayaux, M. J. (1982). Female fecundity as a function of age. *New England Journal of Medicine*, **306**, 404–6.

Federation CECOS, Le Lannou, D. & Lansac, J. (1989). Artificial procreation with frozen donor semen: experience of the French Federation CECOS. *Human Reproduction*, **4**, 757–61.

Forse, R. A., Ackman, C. F. D. & Fraser, F. C. (1985). Possible teratogenic effects of artificial insemination by donor. *Clinical Genetics*, **28**, 23–6.

Jalbert, P., Leonard, C., Selva, J. & David, G. (1989) Genetic aspects of artificial insemination with donor semen: the French CECOS Federation guidelines. *American Journal of Genetics*, **33**, 269–75.

Lansac, J., Le Lannou, D., Imbault, M., Motreff, M:, Lecomte, C. et Prot, C. (1984). La grossesse et l'accouchement après insemination avec du sperme congèle de donneur. *Rev. fr. Gynecol. Obstet.*, **79**, 565–70.

Le Lannou, D., Lobcl, B. & Chambon, Y. (1980). Sperm bank and donor recruitment in France. In *Human Insemination and Semen Preservation*. David G. & Price W. S. eds. pp. 89–94, New York and London: Plenum Press.

Le Lannou, D., Laroche, M., Omnie-bie, M., Gastard, E., Goeho, A., Sevene, L. & Reyes, C. (1989). Intérèts des inséminations intra utérines dans un programme d'IAD. *Contraception, Fertility and Sterility*, **17**, 665–6.

Le Lannou, D., Gastard, E., Gueho, A., Lecalve, M., Lescoat, D., Grall, J.Y., Poulain, P., Giraud, J. R. & Reyes, C. (1990). Les procréations artificielles avec sperme congèle de donneurs. *Contraception, Fertility, Sexuality*, **18**, 601–2.

Richter, M., Haning, R. V. & Chapiro, S. (1984). Artificial donor insemination: fresh versus frozen semen; the patient has her own control. *Fertility and Sterility*, **41**, 277–80.

Schwartz, D. & Mayaux, M. J. (1980). Mode of evaluation of results in artificial insemination. In: *Human Artificial Insemination and Semen Preservation*. David, G. & Price, W .S. eds., pp. 197–200, Plenum Press New York and London.

Selva, J., Leonard, C., Albert, M., Auger, J. & David, G. (1986). Genetic screening for artificial insemination by donors. *Clinics in Genetics*, **29**, 81–8.

Smith, K. D., Rodriguez-Rigau, L. J. & Steinberger, E. (1981). The influence of ovulatory dysfunction and timing of insemination on the success of artificial insemination donor with fresh or cryopreserved semen. *Fertility and Sterility*, **36**, 496–502.

Steinberger, E. & Smith, K.D. (1973). Artificial insemination with fresh and frozen semen: a comparative study. *Journal of the American Medical Association*, **223**, 778–81.

Trounson, A. O., Mahadevan, M., Wood, J. & Leeton, J. F. (1979). Studies on the deep-freezing and artificial insemination of human semen. In

Frozen Human Semen, Richardson D., Joyce D. & Symonds M., eds., pp. 173–183, London: Royal College of Obstetricians and Gynaecologists.

Trounson, A. O., Matthews, C. D., Kovacs, G. T., Spiers, A., Steigrad, S. J., Saunders, D. M., Jones, W. R. & Fuller, S. (1981). Artificial insemination by frozen donor semen: results of multicentre Australian experience. *International Journal of Andrology*, **4**, 227–32.

12

Statistical analysis of data

E. J. LAMB

Basic statistical terms

Analysis of donor insemination data is best done by survival analysis methods based on life tables or the Cox model. Since most readers of this chapter are not statisticians, this discussion will be intuitive and, to the greatest extent possible, not mathematical. Before taking on these relatively complex methods, methods of analysis for studies in which repeated trials, missing data, and changes with time play no role will be reviewed (Table 12.1).

The 2 × 2 contingency table

Results of many comparative studies can be displayed in a 2 × 2 contingency table (Table 12.1). The author finds it helpful to follow certain conventions in constructing these tables. Data for the independent variable – which can be any characteristic of the subject, treatment, test result, or risk factor – are arranged by rows that are labelled on the left. The dependent variable data, arranged by columns labelled on top, can be any event or condition. For donor insemination, the condition is pregnancy and the 'gold standard test' for its presence may be the pregnancy test or clinical examination (Table 12.2).

When analysing data from the medical literature, one must pay attention to rearranging the data in a consistent manner since these conventions are not followed regularly by all authors. A microcomputer spreadsheet, such as Lotus 1-2-3 (Lotus Development Corporation, 1985), programmed to calculate the formulae shown in Fig. 12.1 is a very useful aid. The data entry screen, shown in the top part of Table 12.2,

Table 12.1. *The two by two contingency table, conventions and formulae*

		Condition	
		+ A	− B
Characteristic	+		
	−	C	D

The risk ratio (relative risk of occurrence) = $[A/(A + B)]/[C/(C + D)]$
The odds ratio (relative risk of exposure) = $(A/C)/(B/D)$
Chi square = $\Sigma[(O − E)^2/E]$
Chi square = $[(A + B + C + D)(AD − BC)^2]/[(A + B)(C + D)(A + C)(B + D)]$
Sensitivity = $A/(A + C)$

Specificity = $D/(D + B)$

Positive predictive value = $A/(A + B)$
Negative predictive value = $D/(C + D)$

Positive likelihood ratio = $[A/(A + C)]/[B/(B + D)]$
Negative likelihood ratio = $[C/(A + C)]/[D/(B + D)]$

Table 12.2. *Use of the two by two contingency table*

Source: Fictitious data
Condition: Pregnancy
Test +: New method for insemination

		Condition		
		+	−	Total
Characteristic	+	62	38	100
	−	50	50	100
Total		112	88	200

Risk ratio	1.24	
Odds ratio	1.63	
Chi square	2.92	If chi square $> = 3.84$, $P < = 0.05$
With correction	2.45	If chi square $> = 6.63$, $P < = 0.01$

should have space for recording the source of the data and should force the analyst to make an explicit statement of what is meant by 'positive' for the condition and what is meant by a 'positive' characteristic or test result. The formulae in Table 12.1 for calculating sensitivity, specificity, predictive values, and likelihood ratios are relevant primarily when the independent variable is a laboratory test (Polanksy & Lamb, 1989) and will not be discussed in this review.

Relative risk

Relative risk, a convenient summary of results, may be calculated as one of two different ratios. The risk ratio is the ratio of the rate at which the condition or event occurs among people having the characteristic divided by the rate at which it occurs in those without it. In Table 12.2, the risk ratio of 1.24 was determined as the ratio of the proportion of pregnancy among those treated with the new method (62 of 100 or .620) to the proportion among the controls (50 of 100 or .500). A ratio above one means that the group positive for the characteristic, the new treatment, had a greater chance of having a pregnancy. A ratio of one would mean equal risks for each group and a ratio below one would mean a lower risk for the positive, new treatment, group.

For case control studies, the investigator collects data regarding two groups, the cases, who are people with the disease, and the controls, who are people free of the disease. The investigator starts with a group of cases and selects one or more controls for each case. For example, if an investigator were to select from a database 100 couples who have conceived in the first cycle and then, from among those who have not conceived in that cycle, were to select for each case a control couple matched on the basis of the woman's age, then it would be a case control study. The study might compare how many in each group had used intrauterine and how many had used intracervical insemination.

Important to the analysis of a case control study is the fact that the investigator determines how many are in each group. Because the right hand marginal totals used in calculating risk ratios are under control of the investigator, a different ratio that does not use these marginal totals must be used to estimate the relative risk in case control studies. The formula for this ratio, called the odds ratio, is given in Table 12.1. The analyst must be aware of which is the appropriate ratio to use since the results of the calculations may differ considerably.

Significance level

The risk ratio in Table 12.2 tells us that the group treated with the new method became pregnant 24% more frequently than the control group. At least two possible reasons must be considered: 1) the new method had a real effect on outcome, or 2) the group treated by the new method by chance contained disproportionately many women who would have become pregnant anyway. The fundamental question to ask is this: is a risk ratio of 1.24 significantly different from 1 for a study of this size? The null hypothesis, that the test result has no effect on the presence of the condition and that the results observed occurred by chance variation alone, can be subjected to statistical testing. For data which can be displayed in a 2×2 table, the statistical test of whether the relative risk differs from one is the chi-square (χ^2) test. By use of the chi-square test, one can calculate the probability, P, of getting by chance alone a difference at least as large as that observed if the two groups were, in fact, equivalent. In this statement of probability, P is the significance level.

The chi-square test

The data used to calculate the chi-square test statistic are the observed number (O) and the expected number (E) in each of the four cells A, B, C, D. If the null hypothesis were true, one would expect to have pregnancies among the women treated with the new method in about the same proportion as was found for the total group, that is 112/200 or 56%. Thus one would expect 56 of the 100 women treated with the new method to have conceived. The difference between the observed and the expected number ($O–E$) for cell A is 62 minus 56 or 6. The value of ($O–E$)^2 can be determined for each cell and the chi-square statistic obtained using the first chi-square formula in Table 12.1. For manual of spread-sheet calculations, however, the mathematically equivalent second formula is easier.

The chi-square result calculated from the data in Table 12.2 is compared with the two values of interest extracted from a table of the chi-square distribution with one degree of freedom. We see that a chi-square value of 2.92 is less than that required for statistical significance at the 0.05 level. The difference is not statistically significant at this level. This means that, if there were no difference between the effects of the two treatments and the only cause of differences in outcome between the treatment groups were a chance allocation of more good prognosis patients to one group than to the other, the chance of one treatment group faring at least this much better than the other group would be more than 0.05, that is, more than 1 chance in 20.

Since cells A, B, C, and D each contained at least 20, this method of calculation of our two by two table is applicable. For smaller groups, a corrected chi-square statistic could be calculated or the Fisher exact test used. It is not necessary to review these tests, which the reader will find in statistics texts, to understand the concepts developed later in this chapter.

Alpha and beta errors

Two types of errors are possible in decisions about the null hypothesis. A type I error, rejecting the null hypothesis as false when it is really true, results in attributing to the character or treatment an effect that it really does not have. The probability of erring in this way is indicated by α. Accepting a false null hypothesis, that is deciding that no significant difference exists when there is a real difference in the effectiveness of treatments, is a type II error, and the probability of erring in this way is indicated by β. The probability of disclosing a difference when one actually exists $(1 - \beta)$ is called the power of the statistical test.

Confidence intervals

Reporting the P value alone directs all attention to one boundary of the confidence interval. Reporting the full confidence interval provides much more useful information. The difference between treatments is significant if the 95% confidence interval does not include a relative risk of 1. It is a mistake to consider the identity of two treatments proven when no significant difference can be shown. Many trials end with a finding of no-difference-from-control because the sample size was not adequate. Therapies with clinically meaningful effects may be discarded as ineffective after negative trials that included too few people. If the confidence interval includes the possibility of a strong effect, the study should not be classified as simply a negative study (Freiman *et al.*, 1978).

Randomized clinical trial

An investigator wishing to evaluate a new regimen might first consider placing all subjects on the study regimen and comparing the outcomes with those obtained with subjects previously treated in a similar setting using the standard regimen. This design, using historical controls, is common in exploratory, retrospective studies. However, the advantage of having larger numbers in both groups is more than offset by the strong possibility that systematic differences exist between the groups. These differences are so great that an effect detected at the 5% significance level is often not convincing to those who carefully read the report. Unless an experiment is constructed in a way that a valid estimate of error is possible, it will prove nothing. The process of randomization and the rest of the elaborate precautions to avoid systematic sources of error are necessary to allow statistical evaluation. The randomized clinical trial, a prospective controlled experiment in which the therapies under study are allocated by a chance mechanism, is the most effective way of determining the relative efficacy and hazards of a new therapy.

Balance and stratification

Information about the indication for insemination (azoospermia, oligospermia, etc.), the age and parity of the female, and other factors that might affect prognosis, such as the presence of endometriosis, tubal disease, or ovulation disorders (Collins *et al.*, 1984, Chauhan *et al.*, 1989) should be recorded for all subjects prior to their entry into the study. For each insemination cycle, other factors that should be recorded include the method of cryopreservation, the post-thaw count and motility, the number of inseminations in the cycle, and the method of monitoring ovulation. A relational database is most helpful for recording and analysing such information. So long as their assignment to treatment groups is random, it is unnecessary to balance the number of subjects admitted to the study who show various characteristics which may be prognostic variables.

Retrospective stratification to detect and correct for the effect of these covariates can be done during analysis of the data using the methods discussed later in this chapter (Peto *et al.*, 1976).

Making the first estimate of sample size

During the planning phase, before initiating the trial, one can determine whether there is a reasonable chance of obtaining definitive results by addressing a few questions. 1) What cumulative probability of pregnancy, P_1, do you expect at the time of analysis for the control group? 2) What cumulative probability of pregnancy, P_2, do you expect for the treatment group given the greatest plausible effectiveness of the treatment? 3) How many patients can you reasonably expect to randomize into the study per year? 4) What level of assurance (1 minus α), do you require that you will not report a difference due merely to chance? 5) What level of assurance (1 minus β) do you need that you will not miss a real difference in effectiveness of the treatment?

If other conditions are the same, as β increases, α decreases and vice versa. The probability of making an error of either the first or the second kind is decreased by increasing the sample size. From standard formulae in textbooks one can determine the number of observations required to attain a certain level of assurance $(1 - \beta)$ of demonstrating a significant (α) difference in the outcome of two treatments with true event rates of P_1 and P_2. In practice, the value set for probability α is almost always 0.05 and that for β 0.10 or 0.20. Tables for estimating sample size for comparison of two groups using a binary end point, such as pregnant or not, are found in most introductory statistics texts and in the specialized text by Fleiss on the analysis of rates and proportions (Fleiss, 1981). A most helpful initial approach is to use a graph such as Fig. 12.1 (Feigl, 1978) to determine what difference, $(P_1 - P_2)$, the study can detect for a fixed α and β if n patients are entered per treatment group. Similarly, when the feasible sample size is known, the detectable difference can be read directly from the graph (Fig. 12.1).

As an example, consider clinicians who wish to evaluate a new technique for donor insemination. They expect the cumulative probability of pregnancy, P_1, at the time of evaluation after six cycles of standard treatment, to be 45%. They think it would be feasible to enter about 200 patients during a three year period, enough for 100 in each group, new and standard. They want to have an 80% level of assurance that they will not miss a real improvement in effectiveness ($\beta = 0.20$) and they plan to test at the 5% level of significance ($\alpha = 0.05$) in a one-sided test. From Fig. 12.1 we see that, if P_1 is 0.45 and n is 100, the minimum difference (P_2 minus P_1) must be approximately 0.18. In other words, the cumulative probability of pregnancy at the time of analysis for the treatment group must be greater than 63 to attain statistical significance.

If it seems unreasonable that this cumulative probability could be achieved, a change in one of the elements in the analysis is required. It should be neither the significance level, $P = 0.05$, nor the estimate of the probability of pregnancy with the standard method if that estimate were based on reasonable evidence. Use of a more liberal β should be done

N = number of observations <u>per group</u>

δ = $P_2 - P_1$ = difference to be detected

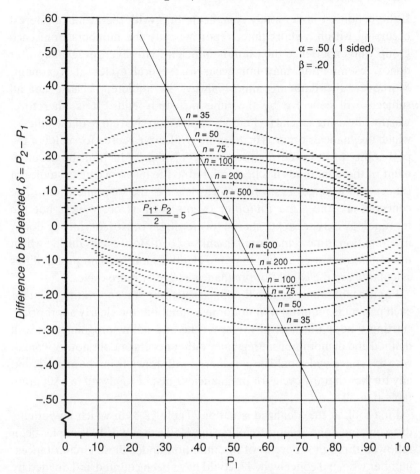

Fig. 12.1. This nomogram can be used to estimate the sample sizes required for testing two independent proportions, P_1 and P_2, with 80% probability of obtaining a significant result at the 5% level. Nomograms for other levels of alpha and beta are given in the original article. Reprinted from Feigl, 1978 with permission.

consciously and only after careful consideration. If the decision is made to proceed with the study, the best approach is to increase the sample size by prolonging the intake period or by enlisting the collaboration of other investigators.

Survival analysis methods

Survival curves

If the condition under study is an acute one, with the event of interest occurring within a short time, reporting only the numbers from each group who experience the event is sufficient. However, pregnancy after donor insemination may not occur for several cycles of treatment. Moreover, the data are almost always incomplete, because not all subjects will conceive by the time the study ends. It is, therefore, worthwhile using special techniques to plot a survival curve of the times at which pregnancies occur. The term survival curve is used for a plot of the probability of the event in question versus time. Much of the development of these methods has been related to life insurance or to studies of cancer and other diseases for which death is the outcome event. The concepts are the same for other events such as pregnancy, but the terminology may seem peculiar in this setting. For patients having donor insemination, time is measured in units of ovulatory cycles during which insemination is used rather than in calendar months. The probabilities calculated are the chance of pregnancy in one or more cycles.

For life table analysis, a well-defined starting point and ending point for each patient is required. For donor insemination, the clearly appropriate starting time is the start of therapy. The end point, pregnancy, is well defined and dichotomous; pregnancy either occurs or does not. A woman who has conceived should be considered withdrawn from the analysis and any further therapy cycles or pregnancies must be analysed in a separate table if at all.

First look at the idealized situation, Table 12.3, in which no patients drop out and none are lost to follow up. Had a group of 100 couples been followed through six cycles of insemination under these circumstances, number who had conceived, 47, could have been counted and divided by 100 to determine the overall probability of conception. Unfortunately, this method of calculation is frequently reported in comparative studies of donor insemination in which the result has much less meaning because of the presence of losses and drop-outs.

Conditional probability of pregnancy

From the data in Table 12.3, the conditional probability of pregnancy can be calculated, that is the probability of conception during an interval for those who have survived the preceding interval without pregnancy. To

Table 12.3. *Life table estimates of conceptions for one group with no loss to follow-up or other censored data*

Cycle	Number treated	Number of terminations		Conditional probability of pregnancy during cycle[a]	Cumulative probability of pregnancy by end of cycle[b]
		Pregnancy	Censored		
1	100	10	0	0.100	0.100
2	90	9	0	0.100	0.190
3	81	8	0	0.099	0.270
4	73	7	0	0.096	0.340
5	66	7	0	0.106	0.410
6	59	6	0	0.102	0.470
Total	469	47			

[a] Conditional probability of pregnancy in cycle n = number pregnant/number treated in cycle n.

[b] Cumulative probability of pregnancy in cycle n = cumulative probability of pregnancy in the previous cycle $(n - 1)$ plus conditional probability of pregnancy in cycle n times the cumulative proportion not pregnant. The cumulative proportion not pregnant is one minus the cumulative probability of pregnancy at the end of the previous cycle.

conceive during the second cycle, a patient must not have conceived during the first. Of the 90 at risk at the beginning of the second cycle, nine conceive and thus the conditional probability of pregnancy in the second cycle is 0.100. These nine are not treated in the third cycle. Of the remaining 81 at risk, eight conceive, giving a conditional probability for that cycle of 0.099. The conditional probability of pregnancy during any cycle is obtained by dividing the number of subjects who became pregnant by the number treated in that cycle. This monthly conditional probability of pregnancy is termed fecundability or fecundity.

The cumulative probability of pregnancy

For the second cycle, one multiplies the conditional probability of pregnancy during the cycle, 0.100, by the cumulative proportion not pregnant at the start of that cycle, that is by one minus the cumulative probability of pregnancy at the end of the previous cycle, $(1 - 0.100)$. Adding the product to the cumulative probability of pregnancy for the preceding cycle, one obtains the cumulative probability at the end of the second cycle: 0.100 plus 0.090 or 0.190. The process is repeated for each succeeding cycle, as shown in Table 12.3, to obtain data for the entire survival curve.

Censored observations

In practice, we do not have a single group of patients all of whom have been continually followed for the same period of time. Patients enter the study one by one. Some become pregnant and others, having survived in the non-pregnant state after a certain number of treatment cycles, stop treatment, are lost to follow-up, or continue in treatment at the time of the analysis. All of these situations in which the patient is no longer exposed to the risk of pregnancy or in which information is lacked about the patient's status, yield incomplete observations called censored observations. Life table methods use all available follow-up information, including censored observations, and thus are more efficient and less subject to error due to incomplete follow-up than direct calculations.

Methods of analysis

Average monthly fecundability: the single parameter model

Assuming that fecundability is relatively constant, a good estimate of the average monthly fecundability is obtained by dividing the number of pregnancies observed by the sum of the person–months of exposure over all intervals (Cramer, Walker & Schiff, 1979). Use of this $\hat{f}$ statistic is appealing because of its computational and interpretive simplicity. It corrects for the presence of censored observations and for non-standard intervals of follow-up.

$$\hat{f} = \Sigma C_i / \Sigma T_i \tag{1}$$

The totals ΣC_6 and ΣT_6 are shown in the last line of Tables 12.3 and 12.4. In Table 12.3, $\hat{f} = 47/469$ or 0.100. In Table 12.4, for the standard method $\hat{f} = 47/442$ or 0.106 and for the new method $\hat{f} = 59/408$ or 0.145.

This estimate of average monthly fecundability is based upon a mathematical model of infertility which assumes that the distribution of conceptions over time is an exponential or geometric one. Such a distribution can be described by a single parameter, the hazard rate, which is constant over the time interval studied. In this case, it is assumed that the couple's hazard rate for pregnancy, their monthly fecundability,

f, remains constant until conception is achieved. To assume constant fecundability is to say that, within the time span studied, pregnancies occur in a random pattern in those at risk, influenced neither by memory of past events nor by the cycle of treatment (Fig. 12.2).

The assumption of a constant hazard rate in survival analysis results in mathematical features which make its use appealing. For instance, the cumulative probability of pregnancy when plotted against treatment cycles has a smooth exponential increase, Fig. 12.2. Pregnancy is a positive event and an ascending curve of this type is most often used in studies of donor insemination.

Assuming that all women in the cohort would eventually conceive, the mean interval to conception has a simple reciprocal relationship with fecundability.

$$MIC = 1/f \tag{2}$$

The cumulative probability of pregnancy at time t can be estimated by:

$$P = 1 - (1 - f)^t \tag{3}$$

or

$$P = 1 - \exp(-ft) \tag{4}$$

If only a graphic representation of the life table is published, one can make an estimate of the average fecundability by reading the cumulative probability of pregnancy at several times, t, on the curve and applying the following formula:

$$f = (1 - P)^{1/t} \tag{5}$$

Cramer gives a method to calculate the confidence limits of $\hat{f}$ based upon the assumption that conceptions are distributed over the period of time as a Poisson variable (Cramer *et al.*, 1979).

$$\frac{\Sigma C_i \pm 1.96\sqrt{\Sigma C_i}}{\Sigma T_i} = \begin{cases} \dfrac{47 + 1.96\sqrt{47}}{442} - 0.137 \\[2ex] \dfrac{47 - 1.96\sqrt{47}}{442} = 0.076 \end{cases} \tag{6}$$

For the standard method in Table 12.4, for example, with $\hat{f}$ of 0.106, the 95% confidence limits would be $(47 \pm (1.96 \times \sqrt{47}))/\sqrt{442}$ or

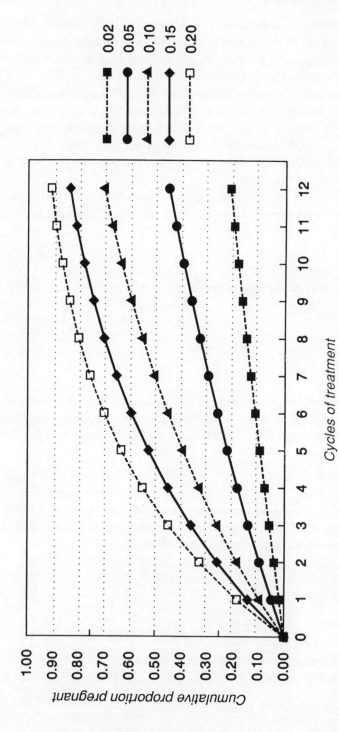

Fig. 12.2. This family of curves illustrates the cumulative proportion of conceptions at end of cycles 1 through 12 obtained with various constant fecundabilities, f. An f of .02 is typical for an infertility clinic population. By the end of 5 years at this f, 70% will have become pregnant. An f of .10 is typical of results of donor insemination programs. An f of .20 is considered normal fertility.

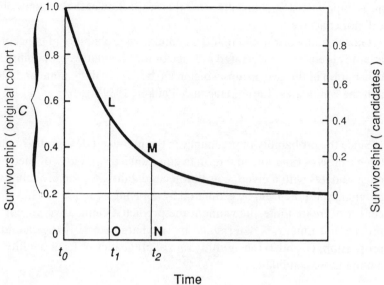

Fig. 12.3.

.076 to .137. Other methods of determining confidence limits are discussed by Higgins and Wilkins, 1985.

This single parameter, or constant hazard rate, model has been widely applied in studies of donor insemination. Fortunately, the hazard rate, as determined by the monthly conditional probability of conception calculated in life tables, is fairly constant. When this conditional probability is plotted against time, the slope of the line does not usually differ significantly from 0, at least when the partner in the infertile marriage has azoospermia. When the slope deviates from zero, one must consider the possibility that some of the female recipients have characteristics which markedly reduce their fecundability.

The two parameter model: candidates and non-candidates

Guzick and Rock demonstrated that fecundability calculated this way for a group of women surgically treated for endometriosis was not constant but declined with time (Guzick & Rock, 1981). They postulated, as one possible model to reconcile their findings, that some women are actually never going to conceive following therapy but are, in fact, covertly sterile. In Fig. 12.3, survivorship in the not-pregnant state $(1 - P)$ is plotted against cycles of treatment giving a declining exponential curve reaching an asymptote at 0.20, indicating that this proportion of the original cohort will not conceive.

Guzick and Rock noted that the cumulative probability of conception at time t is equal to a weighted average of the cumulative probabilities of conception in the two groups which have been called the non-candidates and the candidates (Lamb, Hagen & Pauker, 1989):

$$P_t = (1 - C) \cdot P_{t,\text{not}-C} + C \cdot P_{t,C} \tag{7}$$

Since the probability of pregnancy in the non-candidate group remains 0 regardless of time, the first term in equation 3 drops out. For the group of candidates with a given, constant fecundability, f_C, the probability of pregnancy at time t can be estimated by applying equation 4. Thus, for a cohort of treated infertile women, the predicted cumulative proportion pregnant at time, t, is determined by two parameters: 1) the candidacy proportion, C, and 2) the monthly rate of pregnancy or fecundability, f_C, among those candidates:

$$P_{t,C} = 1 - \exp(-f_C \cdot t) \tag{8}$$

The mean interval of observation, MIO, between times t_1 and t_2 is represented by the area of the polygon LMNO. The proportion of non-candidates in the total cohort is larger in this interval than in any earlier interval and smaller than in any subsequent interval. Were fecundability estimated using MIO in place of MIC, the mean interval to conception, in equation 2, fecundability would appear to progressively decline with time. The fecundability of the candidate group, however, is constant as shown by the declining exponential curve reaching an asymptote at $(1 - C)$, 0.20 in this example.

This two parameter model requires a microcomputer for calculation of the candidacy proportion, C. It has been applied to studies of donor insemination (Peek et al., 1984; Bradshaw, Guzik, Grun et al., 1987) and to formal decision analysis of infertility (Lamb, Hagen, & Pauker, 1989). A similar approach must be taken for analysing survival after treatment of such tumors as lymphoma where cure is common and the hazard rate for death among non-cured patients appears to be constant (Berkson & Cage, 1952).

Life table analysis with censored observations

In Table 12.4, we have used fictitious data to illustrate the life table method of calculating the cumulative probability of pregnancy when

Table 12.4. *Life table estimates of pregnancy for two groups (some censored observations in both groups)*

Cycle	Number treated	Number of terminations		Conditional probability of pregnancy during cycle[a]	Cumulative probability of pregnancy by end of cycle[b]
		Pregnancy	Censored		
Standard method					
1	100	10	1	0.100	0.100
2	89	9	3	0.101	0.191
3	77	8	1	0.104	0.275
4	68	7	2	0.103	0.350
5	59	7	3	0.119	0.427
6	49	6	43	0.122	0.497
Total	442	47			
New method					
1	100	15	1	0.150	0.150
2	84	10	3	0.143	0.271
3	71	9	1	0.159	0.388
4	61	8	2	0.140	0.474
5	51	7	3	0.146	0.550
6	41	7	34	0.150	0.618
Total	398	59			

[a,b] See footnotes to Table 12.3.

there are censored observations. As before, the number treated at the start of each cycle is obtained by subtracting from the number at risk at the beginning of the preceding cycle the number who conceived or terminated for other reasons during the preceding cycle. For example, at the start of cycle 2 of the standard treatment, only 89 of the original 100 are still at risk. The proportion of conceptions during the cycle is obtained by dividing the number of conceptions during the cycle by the number treated: 9/89 = 0.101. Although the conditional probability of pregnancy is constant from cycle to cycle in this example, life table analysis does not assume a constant fecundability or any specific distribution of pregnancies with time.

In life table calculations, censored observations are not ignored but influence the calculated rates only in so far as the information is available. Thus, these methods allow maximum utilization of information. The cumulative probabilities so determined allow one to compare groups that vary in size, in relative magnitude of the conditional probability of pregnancy in various cycles, and in completeness of follow-up. These methods allow comparison with the conception curve for a control group or for the general population.

The method most commonly used today, because of the ready availability of microcomputers, examines individual survival times and is called the product limit method (Kaplan & Meier, 1958). The actuarial life table estimate (Cutler & Ederer, 1958; Lamb & Cruz, 1972, Cooke *et al.*, 1981) which groups data by time intervals may be used for manual calculations. When the Cutler–Ederer actuarial method is used, events can occur at various times during an interval and the effective number exposed to the risk during the interval is calculated by subtracting one-half of the pregnancies and censored observations occurring during the interval from the number at risk at the start of the interval. This is based on the assumption that registration and the censoring events are roughly equally distributed during the interval. Thus one assumes that people are exposed to the risk for half the interval on the average. This correction does not apply to the risks of conception during a single treatment cycle of insemination and should not be used when data are displayed as shown in Table 12.4.

Comparison of two survival curves

Log-rank analysis of differences in a single variable

The statistical method used in comparison of two survival curves is one based upon the chi-square test. Imagine constructing a 2×2 contingency table comparing the two groups at every point on the life table graph at which a pregnancy occurs. From the observed and the expected number in each of the four cells, A, B, C, and D, the chi-square statistic can be calculated for that interval. Now, if the observation window is passed across the entire life table graph from the beginning, stopping to accumulate the chi-square statistics on the way, a summary chi-square statistic is derived, a measure of the significance of the difference between the two curves.

This summary chi-square technique is called the Mantel–Haenszel method of log-rank analysis (Mantel, 1966). Using the Mantel–Haenszel technique, it is possible to compare the probability of conception among two or more treatment groups. Because the chi-square statistics are added, it is possible to adjust by stratification during analysis for differences among subgroups to control for relevant prognostic factors such as

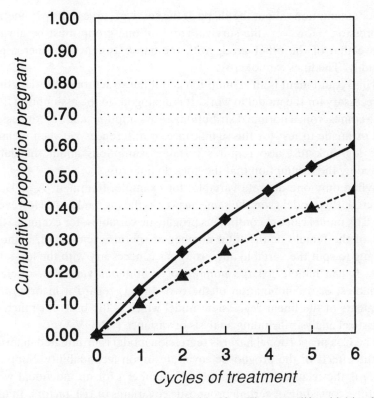

Fig. 12.4. Graphic life table of data of Table 12.4. The term 'life table' is often used to refer to a graph such as this.

age or stage of disease (Peto *et al.*, 1977). An overall estimate of the relative effects of treatments A and B adjusted for each of the initial prognostic factors is obtained.

Cox proportional hazards model

The potential predictors identified by log-rank analysis may be entered into a multiple variable analysis by means of the proportional hazards model introduced by Cox (Cox, 1972). This multiple regression technique is a generalization of the log-rank test. It assumes that the hazard rates, fecundabilities, are proportional among the groups analysed. This means that the relative risk associated with a given level of the prognostic variable does not change with time. Thus it is called the proportional hazard regression model. It requires neither a constant hazard rate nor other assumptions about the shape of the survival curve or its parametric expression. However, the survival curve of one group must be always above that of the other group with the gap between them increasing steadily. The lines cannot cross.

This requirement is an assumption about the structure of the data that is necessary for the model to work. It is analogous to the assumption that data comes from a normal distribution, an assumption made before using the t-statistic to test for the significance of differences between means. The log-rank test also requires certain assumptions about the data, including the assumption that the lines do not cross.

When only one discrete variable, for example, treatment A or B, is entered, this model gives the same answer as the log-rank test. However, the Cox model can use continuous prognostic variables, for example, the age of the female or the total number of sperm inseminated, without having to split the variable into groups as is necessary with the log-rank test. It can handle a large number of continuous variables, discrete variables, or a combination of the two. In this regard it incorporates elements of the linear regression model which is the basis for much of statistical analysis including analysis of variance (ANOVA).

The Cox proportional hazards regression model is formulated in terms of the effects of the prognostic covariates upon fecundability. Suppose $f(t;z)$ is the fecundability during cycle number t for an individual with vector z consisting of certain prognostic covariates or risk factors. In this example, the individual might be a woman of age 35 receiving 40 million sperm by intrauterine insemination. The proportional hazard model is given by:

$$f(t;z) = f_o(t) \exp(\beta z) \tag{9}$$

or the mathematically equivalent:

$$f(t;z) = f_o(t)(e^\beta)^z \tag{10}$$

where β is a vector of unknown regression coefficients and $f_o(t)$ is an unknown fecundability at time t for an individual with the covariate vector z equal to 0.

In this example, the individual might be age 20, the youngest in the study, receiving 5 million sperm, the lowest number in the study, by inter-cervical insemination, the method assigned a value of 0, intrauterine being assigned a value of 1. The term e^β, the conversion factor, relates the effect of covariate on fecundability. In studies of survival from disease, it is called the excess mortality factor. In the current setting, think of e^β as the conception factor. The e^{β} statistic, has a value between 0 and infinity. A value of 1.0 means that the characteristic has no influence on the rate of subsequent conception. A value of <1.0 indicates a progressive decrease in conception rates with increases in the value of a given variable over its entire distribution and an estimate >1.0 indicates an increase in the rate of conception. The further away from unity, the stronger the influence. A summary chi-square statistic is used to test the null hypothesis that the conception factor equals 1.0.

The paper by Cox is difficult for those who are not mathematicians. Fortunately, explanations more complete than this chapter that are still intuitive may be found in Peto *et al.*, 1976 and in Tibshirani, 1982. A more complete exposition is found in Lee, 1980.

Estimation of sample size

In survival analysis, calculation of appropriate sample size is more difficult than that previously outlined as a first approximation. The dependent variable for analysis is the time to conception rather than the binary variable, pregnant-or-not which applied in the method of sample size calculation previously outlined as a first approximation. For a survival analysis study with a given annual rate of entry of subjects and predetermined values for α and β the question of sample size can be translated into a question of the required length of accrual and follow-up. A microcomputer program is available which can interactively determine the most desirable combination of accrual and follow-up times using Monte Carlo simulations (Halpern & Brown, 1987). This program can also accommodate various proportions of candidates and non-candidates as well as arbitrary shapes of the survival curves, even estimates hand drawn by the investigator.

A crossover design is popular in studies of methods used for donor insemination. Typically, treatment given in the first cycle is assigned by a random process and the standard and new methods used in alternating cycles thereafter. Data from the two treatments A and B, have been analysed as independent survival curves (Cooke *et al.*, 1981).

A better approach would be to use the data on each woman as a single observation and regard the procedure, A or B, as a time dependent covariate in a Cox proportional hazards analysis.

Since, in general, smaller sample sizes are needed for crossover designs, estimates of sample size made by one of the methods previously mentioned may be considered conservative if a cross-over design is used.

Complete analysis of insemination data

Complete analysis of donor insemination data includes three steps: 1) organization of follow-up data in a life table, 2) analysis of single variable differences, for example, treatment and control groups, by log-rank tests, and 3) analysis of multiple variables by use of the Cox proportional hazards regression model.

Only a few data items need be tabulated for the application of these methods: an identification number for each patient, treatment group (new method or standard), cycle number of treatment, and outcome (pregnant or not). In addition, data regarding other prognostic variables must be tabulated if the Cox proportional hazards regression model is to be used. Although the calculations for life tables can be done by hand using the formulae in Table 12.3, a spreadsheet program such as Lotus 1-2-3 (Lotus Development Corporation) is most helpful. Special statistical computer programs are necessary for the two-parameter model (Guzick & Rock, 1981, Lamb, Hagen & Pauker, 1989) and for the Cox model (Dixon *et al.*, 1983).

In 1976, the Medical Research Council published a clear succinct report written by ten experienced statisticians specifically to give physicians the statistical ideas and methods needed to design, carry out, and analyse clinical trials (Peto *et al.*, 1976, 1977). The report avoids statistical jargon, provides all necessary tables, and provides worked examples. It remains the single best sources of information for the non-statistician interested in learning the techniques of survival analysis including the Cox model. Although the examples are from oncology trials, the basic concepts are readily applied to donor insemination studies.

The proportional hazards model represents the state of the art in analysis of insemination data. By including within the model a number of prognostic variables, it provides the most sensitive method to detect differences in effectiveness of two treatment options.

References

Berkson, S. & Gage, R. P. (1952). Survival curve for cancer patients following treatment. *Journal American Statistical Association*, **47**, 501–15.

Bradshaw, K., Guzik, D., Grun, B., Johnson, N. & Ackerman, G. (1987). Cumulative pregnancy rates for donor insemination according to ovulatory function and tubal status. *Fertility and Sterility*, **48**, 1051–4.

Chauhan, M., Barratt, C. L. R., Cooke, S. & Cooke, I. D. (1989). Differences in the fertility of donor insemination recipients. *Fertility and Sterility*, **51**, 815–19.

Collins, J. A., Barner, J. B., Wilson, E. H., Wrixon, W. & Casper, R. F. (1984). A proportional hazards analysis of the clinical characteristics of infertile couples. *American Journal of Obstetrics and Gynecology*, **148**, 527–32.

Cooke, I.D., Sulaiman, R.A., Lenton, E.A. & Parsons, R. J. (1981). Fertility and infertility statistics: their importance and application. *Clinical Obstetrics and Gynaecology*, **8**, 531–48.

Cox, D. R. (1972). Regression models and life-tables. *Journal of the Royal Statistical Society B*, **34**, 187–220.

Cramer, D. W., Walker, A. M. & Schiff, I. (1979). Statistical methods in evaluating the outcome of infertility therapy. *Fertility and Sterility*, **32**, 80–6.

Cutler, S. J. & Ederer, F. (1958). Maximum utilization of the life-table method in analyzing survival. *Journal of Chronic Diseases*, **8**, 699–712.

Dixon, W. J., Brown, W. B., Engleman, L., Frane, J. W., Hill, M. A., Jennrich, R. I. & Toporek, J. D. (1983). *BMDP Statistical Software*, 1983 printing with revisions, Berkeley: University of California Press.

Feigl, P. (1978). A graphical aid for determining sample size when comparing two independent proportions. *Biometrics*, **34**, 111–20.

Fleiss, J. L. (1981). *Statistical Methods for Rates and Proportions*, 2nd edn. John Wiley and Sons, New York.

Freiman, J. A., Chalmers, T. C., Smith, H. & Kuebler, R. R. (1978). The importance of beta, the type II error and sample size in the design and interpretation of the randomized control trial. *New England Journal of Medicine*, **299**, 690–4.

Guzick, D. S. & Rock, J. A. (1981). Estimation of a model of cumulative pregnancy following infertility therapy. *American Journal of Obstetrics and Gynecology*, **140**, 573–8.

Halpern, J. & Brown, B. W. (1987). Cure rate models: power of the log rank and generalized Wilcoxon tests. *Statistics in Medicine*, **6**, 483–9.

Higgins, J. E. & Wilkins, L. R. (1985). Statistical comparison of Pearl rates. *American Journal of Obstetrics and Gynecology*, **151**, 656–9.

Kaplan, E. L. & Meier, P. (1958). Non-parametric estimation from incomplete observations. *Journal of the American Statistical Association*, **53**, 457–81.

Lamb, E. J. & Cruz, A. L. (1972). Data collection and analysis in an infertility practice. *Fertility and Sterility*, **23**, 310–19.

Lamb, E. J., Hagen, M. & Pauker, S. G. (1989). The mean interval to conception: a measure of utility for the analysis of decisions involving fertility. *American Journal of Obstetrics and Gynecology*, **160**, 1470–89.

Lee, E. T. (1980). *Statistical Methods for Survival Data Analysis*. Belmont, CA: Lifetime Learning Publications.

Lotus 1-2-3, version 2.2 (1984). Lotus Development Corporation, Cambridge, MA., 02142, USA.

Mantel, N. (1966). Evaluation of survival data and two new rank order statistics arising in its consideration. *Cancer Chemotherapy Reports*, **50**, 163–71.

Peek, J. (1984). Estimation of fertility in women receiving artifical insemination by donor semen and in normal fertile women. *British Journal of Obstetrics and Gynaecology*, **91**, 1019–24.

Peto, R., Pike, M. C., Armitage, P., Breslow, N. E., Cox, D. R., Howard, S. V., Mantel, N., McPherson, K., Peto, J. & Smith, P. G. (1976). Design and analysis of randomized clinical trials requiring prolonged observation of each patient. I. Introduction and design. *British Journal of Cancer*, **34**, 585–612.

Peto, R., Pike, M. C., Armitage, P., Breslow, N. E., Cox, D. R., Howard, S. V., Mantel, N., McPherson, K., Peto, J. & Smith, P. G. (1977). Design and analysis of randomized clinical trials requiring prolonged observation of each patient. II Analysis and examples. *British Journal of Cancer*, **35**, 1–39.

Polansky, F. F. & Lamb, E. J. (1989). Analysis of three laboratory tests used in evaluation of male fertility. Bayes rule applied to the postcoital test, the *in vitro* mucus migration test and the zona-free hamster egg test. *Fertility and Sterility*, **51**, 215–28.

Tibshirani, R. (1982). A plain man's guide to the proportional hazards model. *Clinical Investigations in Medicine*, **5**, 63–76.

13

Ethical and legal aspects of donor insemination

R. SNOWDEN

This Act of Parliament [The Human Fertilisation and Embryology Act 1990] will regulate embryo research and certain infertility treatments throughout the U.K. It also sets out the legal status of children born as a result of such techniques. In my view it is the most comprehensive measure of this kind in the world.

Kenneth Clarke, Secretary of State for Health, November 1990.

In all actions concerning children, whether undertaken by public or private social welfare institutions, courts of law, administrative authorities or legislative bodies, the best interests of the child shall be the primary consideration.

Article 3, U.N. Convention on the Rights of Children, 1989.

All marital and familial phenomena ultimately come back to connection through birth.

Kingsley Davis, *The Study of Marriage and the Family as a Scientific Discipline.* 1984.

Introduction

The birth of children and their socialization as members of a given society has been, and continues to be, an underlying concern in all societies. The rules by which reproduction and socialization take place may vary between societies and in the same society over time but they are pervasive and more powerful than we often recognize. These rules may be formal and enshrined in law, e.g. proscribed incestuous or under-age sexual relationships or informal but socially enforced by more subtle means, e.g. the selection of 'suitable' marriage partners. The formalization of social rules by means of legislation represents the full extent of the response to

social concern about a particular topic. The earliest expression of such
concern usually takes the form of ethical debate. In most situations a
progression from ethical debate to legislation does not occur because
social concern is insufficiently strong to warrant such regulation but some
topics provoke a demand for legislative control. The creation of children
by the use of semen collected from an anonymous third party is such a
topic. It has taken just over 100 years for donor insemination to be
subjected to this first application of comprehensive legislative control.
Donor insemination is the most common form of assisted conception at
the present time but the need for control of the procedure has doubtless
been accelerated by developments associated with surrogacy arrangements and developments in *in vitro* fertilization and its derivatives. But
why should this particular subject give rise to so much social concern
when all that is being attempted is the alleviation of the frustration of
childlessness among those unfortunately afflicted with infertility?

While not wishing to overstate the case, it is instructive to compare
social interest in the new reproductive techniques with that which took
place in the last century during the debates on evolution. Perhaps this is
the beginning of a debate which encompasses the rights of science at a
time when individual autonomy has taken on the force of ideology
affecting social life at a number of levels. The earlier Darwinian conflicts
– often strongly argued and even now not fully resolved – were associated
with a confrontation between ideological beliefs and rationality which
was popularly seen as a contest between religion and science. The present
ethical debate places science under pressure because the activities undertaken in its name appear to be in conflict with ideological presumptions,
individual human rights and matters of personal identity.

Interference in the human reproductive process is not of itself a matter
of major concern to this debate. There has always been some control over
such matters but this has usually taken the form of pressure associated
with the selection or choice of mate. Examples of what Darwin might call
the 'artificial selection' of a mate among humans are not difficult to find.
The selection of a mate from among a narrowly defined group of those
considered to be socially eligible is an obvious example. In this situation
the 'pedigree' of the resulting child is usually openly noted and often
emphasized. It is not so much the genetic credibility of the child resulting
from donor gametes but the attempts deliberately to obscure such genetic
links which marks out certain of the new assisted conception techniques
as being so contentious. Some clinicians have understood this and are

advocating a greater degree of openness about their work. However, in some respects their endeavours to placate public suspicion have been made more difficult by their success in influencing the content of recent legislation to maintain the anonymity of gamete donors. It seems a situation has been reached where one of the basic tenets of science – that of openness – is being abrogated. Why these questions of secrecy and anonymity should be so important provides the link to the second area of contention which may, in the fullness of time, be regarded as having been the most profoundly affected by gamete donation. This relates to the changes being introduced into those relationships which some would claim are fundamental to personal identity: that is, relationships within the family.

While the ideology of individualism has penetrated social lives – at least in the Western world – there are still those who accept that *who* one is (as distinct from *what* one is) is important and that this sense of identity depends upon those relationships normally associated with parenting and family. This is not to say that these relationships are necessarily good, or successful, or desired, or enjoyed, but they are, nevertheless, important. At one extreme personal identity can be seen as a form of individualism primarily based on biological factors associated with genetic inheritance while at the other extreme such identity is seen as resulting from the relationships formed external to oneself which include those with other people but also with one's general environment. It seems that the nature versus nurture, the genetic versus environmental, the biological versus sociological interpretations of personal identity are resurfacing yet again. It is because of these differing interpretations – and the competition between them – that consideration of the ethical and social complexities attendant upon donor insemination takes the form of an ideological debate with its attendant fervour and disputation. By failing to understand this, those who see such debate as criticism of their own work, and an attack upon medical practice, enter the debate at a different level which allows little opportunity for a meeting of minds.

The importance of family relationships

What makes the study of family relationships so difficult is that the thoughts one brings to bear on such a study have largely been structured by the very relationships being studied. While the thinking content (what is thought about) may be developed or modified as a result of later experience, the structure of such thinking (how one thinks) is likely to be more rigid and enduring and based on early experience. The subject of family relationships is one which is not readily amenable to objective assessment or measurement using the traditional tools of science.

In personal lives people are often made aware of the importance of subjective experiences; indeed it is these positive or negative feelings which tend to have most meaning. While scientific discovery or medical treatment success may be measured in objective terms, it is the subjective sense of exhilaration which follows on from the discovery or success which is so enjoyed. While attempts have been made to scale or measure such subjective feelings, these attempts have not generally succeeded beyond what most would regard as a superficial level. This inability to assess the impact of subjective experiences in ways which permit objective measurement should not be allowed to diminish their significance or lead to an underestimation of their value.*

In terms of relationships with other human beings, it appears that the expression of deepest feelings is normally restricted to a very small number of people. Close family members are usually among the select few who are given the opportunity to see others in ways only permitted by long-term familiarity. The words *family* and *familiar* coming as they do from the same root, emphasize this point. Similarly, the description of certain people as *relatives* signifies the occupation of a special *relationship* with those concerned. It is the subjective and largely immeasurable quality of these relationships which exists between close family relatives that provides such an important dimension to lives. This dimension normally has a past, present and future and is both more sensitive and more enduring the closer the biological relationship. Feelings of pride about the achievements of a son or daughter are usually greater than feelings in response to similar achievements of a niece or nephew.

Family relationships are normally based on biological links. Radcliffe-Brown identified seven *primary* relatives – mother, father, daughter, son, sister, brother, spouse – with *secondary* relatives (primary relatives of ones primary relatives) and *tertiary* relatives (primary relatives of one's secondary relatives) occupying a widening circle of family members. Parents, children and siblings take these biological links within the family for granted; indeed it is likely to be considered improper to question such

---

* The author would argue that the three most important characteristics in determining personal success, namely intelligence, creativity and a desire to achieve, are currently immeasurable in objective terms despite the attempts of psychologists to quantify intelligence as IQ and the achievement motive as *n*Ach.

links. Whilst most relatives share a common biological inheritance, the biological link between spouses is of a different kind. It does not result from a predisposing biological link but one that is created in the future through the combining of their genes in the conception and birth of their own progeny. This distribution of relatives, though biologically based, contains a clear hierarchy of family members attracting differing levels of personal and social rights and duties.

Upon this initial biological link a complex structure of human relationships is built which has considerable psychological and social significance. These special relationships are demonstrated by the commitment family members normally have for each other. Through the socialization process, the internalization of rights and duties lead to the manifestation of individual roles described as those of mother, father, sister, son, etc. which collectively provide the framework for the norms through which social life becomes possible. The expectations underlying all of these processes are the building blocks which allow the transition from a purely biological event when sperm meets egg to eventual active membership of a social group.

Donor insemination erodes the biological links which form the foundations on which family relationships are built. A couple whose child was conceived by donor insemination cannot look at their offspring and see a mingling of their genes; their union has not resulted in the procreation of children. For them, such a child, though much loved, is qualitatively different from a child who is biologically linked to them both and who links them to each other. This has implications for themselves and also for their kinsfolk. If this were not so, the secrecy surrounding the donor insemination procedure, the desire for donor anonymity and the public uncertainty leading to the need for legislation would not have arisen. Reproduction is clearly much more than a biological event.

Public interest in the development of donor insemination services

Public interest in donor insemination was first aroused in the USA following publication of a letter in a medical journal in which the author described an experience which had taken place 25 years earlier (in 1884) during his training as a medical student. This was a case in which a couple were unable to achieve a pregnancy and where the husband was found to be azoospermic. In order to resolve this deficiency of sperms, sperm was 'donated' by a medical student (described as the 'best looking boy in the class') and introduced into the wife while she was under a general anaesthetic. The action, at first, was kept secret from both the husband and wife, but after conception was determined the husband was told, but – at his insistence – not his wife. The secret was kept by all concerned but 25 years later the author of the letter (who had been present in the 1884 class) discreetly enquired after the family and then wrote the letter to the journal. He believed this successful attempt to relieve childlessness had been worthwhile and recommended that donor insemination should be made more widely available.

The reaction to this published account was immediate and prolonged. The topic became a matter of major contention reaching far beyond the medical profession. The ethics of interference with reproduction, the secrecy surrounding the action, the arbitrary nature of the donor selection, the lack of consultation with the couple in advance of treatment and the keeping of knowledge about the child's genetic origins from the child and the child's mother were all hotly debated. Others argued that a procedure such as donor insemination could be used systematically to improve the genetic stock of the population while theologians argued that such a procedure demonstrated a defiance of God and that it was not man's place to create human beings in this way.

This first report includes a number of assumptions which appear to have been accepted throughout the history of donor insemination and other methods of assisted conception. These assumptions underlie most of the uncertainty and contention surrounding these issues; an uncertainty which has become more pronounced with the expansion and improvement of these techniques. The most important assumption is that the act of procreation performed in this way is of purely medical interest and as a consequence only medical considerations concerning the alleviation of the presenting complaint should be considered. Another is that the donation of gametes is of personal concern only, involving the donor without regard to his actual or potential relationships with others or the possible concern of the wider community.

This debate – or series of debates – did not become more than of limited interest in the UK until the mid-1940s when a report appeared in the British Medical Journal which indicated that donor insemination was now being practised in the UK. This report initiated a similar reaction to that experienced three decades earlier in the USA. The most notable contribution to this debate was that made by the Archbishop of Canterbury who believed that legislation should be introduced to make the provision of donor insemination services a criminal offence. The Government reacted slowly to this suggestion and it was not until 1960 that the report of its own inquiry (The Feversham Report) was available. While express-ing disquiet about the social consequences of donor insemination pro-cedures the report did not recommend the introduction of legislation to control such activities. It appeared that the committee members hoped that, by refusing to give legal recognition to donor insemination, couples would be deterred from recourse to such a controversial and unregulated procedure. The Feversham Committee was wrong in this belief for during the 1960s the demand for donor insemination services actually increased. This increase in demand was probably due to the marked reduction in the availability of babies for adoption at a time when abortion became less restrictive and when there was a greater acceptance of single parenthood.

The demand for donor insemination services reached a level which prompted the BMA to set up a working party of its own under the chairmanship of Sir John Peel to study the issue. This reported in 1973 and recommended that such services should be made more widely available under the NHS. This report did not attract as much attention among the general public as previous reports but its impact within the medical profession was significant. It was this report which, in contrast to previous reports, provided professional respectability to the provision of donor insemination services in this country.

Another major impetus to the debates about the availability of donor insemination services came with the birth of the first baby to be born following conception using *in vitro* fertilization in 1978. This birth led to considerable publicity about all assisted conception techniques. As donor insemination was – and continues to be – the most commonly used of these techniques, it is not surprising that it should become, yet again, the subject of discussion and dispute. Following influential media coverage of the new reproductive techniques and the scientific work associated with them, a Committee of Inquiry on Human Fertilization and Embryology was set up by the Government which reported in 1984 (The Warnock Report). Recommendations were made for the regulation of *in vitro* fertilization and donor insemination techniques, for the management of surrogacy arrangements, and for the control of experiments using human embryos. The Warnock Report acted as the basis for the legislation contained in the Human Fertilization and Embryology Act 1990.

The Human Fertilisation and Embryology Act, 1990

This Act is wide ranging and deals with the regulation of a number of topics many of which are indirectly related to donor insemination, e.g.

surrogacy, *in vitro* fertilization using donor gametes, etc. What follows is an outline of the more direct references to donor insemination:

- Setting up of an independent Human Fertilization and Embryology Authority to control and license centres providing donor insemination (and certain other) treatments. This control is exercised through powers given directly by the Act and through a code of practice the Authority is required to develop. While infringement of the code of practice does not, of itself, constitute an offence under the Act, the granting or continuation of the required licence to provide a regulated service may be affected.
- Licences for providing a donor insemination service and for sperm storage must be obtained from the Authority.
- Licences relate to authorized premises with the regulated activities being undertaken under the supervision of a named 'person responsible'.
- Proper records must be maintained at treatment centres concerning person(s) donating or receiving gametes.
- Account must be taken of the welfare of any child who may be born as a result of treatment (including the need of that child for a father) and of any other children who may be affected by the birth.
- Written consent must be obtained from both donor and recipient, and both must be advised of their right to withdraw such consent.
- Both donor and recipient must be given a suitable opportunity to receive proper counselling and must be provided with relevant information relating to the treatment.
- Procedures shall be maintained for determining the persons acting as donors.
- Appropriate storage of sperm must take place.
- The woman who receives the sperm and who carries the child is deemed to be the mother of the child.
- The woman's husband or partner is regarded in all respects as the child's father unless it is shown he did not consent to his partner's insemination.
- Records must be kept by the Authority relating to named donors, those receiving insemination and any resulting child.
- The child has a right to receive certain limited information at the age of 18 years (or earlier in some circumstances) but this does not include the right to knowledge of the identity of the donor at the present time.
- The courts have powers under certain circumstances to demand the name of the donor from the Authority.

Ethical issues still requiring resolution

Even with the presence of the 1990 Act, debate about a number of issues surrounding the provision and use of donor gametes is unlikely to have come to an end. This is partly because the Act has devolved to the new Authority the task of developing a code of practice which is expected to address a number of the unresolved and contentious issues which have been present since 1884 and partly because of the requirements of the Act itself. The code of practice is expected to give guidance about a wide variety of practical issues including such matters as the selection of donors, the number of times a donor should be used and whether or not payment for the purchase of gametes should be permitted. Certain requirements of the Act are also likely to be challenged in the future, especially those dealing with the rights of the child and the stipulation that identifying information about the donor must not be divulged. Space does not permit a detailed listing of all these issues or a full discussion of those selected but the dozen listed below are probably enough to keep the thoughtful observer occupied for some time.

- At what point does medical confidentiality cease and secrecy begin?
- What medical justification is there for treating the fit wife of her infertile husband?
- What medical justification is there for providing donor insemination treatment for a single woman?
- In a society where human tissue and organs are freely donated, is it ethical to allow the sale and purchase of human gametes?
- What is the intended function of donor anonymity?
- Does a person have a right, independently of his existing or future family affiliations, to donate or sell his gametes?
- Should the consent of a potential donor's partner be required?
- Should the donor inform his own children of his activity?
- Who is thought to be protected by donor anonymity – the donor, child, recipient couple, the treatment provider?
- Should the donor be informed of the child's birth?
- How does the legal requirement that account must be taken of the welfare of the child (including the need of that child for a father) affect:
  - (a) the provision of donor insemination services to homosexual individuals or couples;
  - (b) the selection of social parents;
  - (c) the selection of genetic parents;
  - (d) the child's right to relevant information?

- What is the purpose of keeping knowledge of genetic origins from the enquiring child or adult who was conceived by donor insemination?

Conclusion

Legislative interference in medical practice and scientific endeavour inevitably contains a potential for disagreement especially when the protagonists are defending beliefs about such topics as the sanctity of human life, the right to bear children, the rights of children yet to be conceived, the practical problems associated with the treatment of infertility using donated gametes and the freedom surrounding professional judgement. There are still areas of muddle which remain and which legislation is unlikely to resolve. This is mainly because the implications of disconnecting the biological and psychosocial links in family relationships have still to be thought through.

Undoubtedly, donor insemination as a means of alleviating childlessness is here to stay and the Human Fertilization and Embryology Act has been a major step in its management. The most important ethical issues which remain to be resolved are those which relate to the rights and welfare of the planned child. The refusal to allow access to information about a genetic parent when a record of such information exists is an issue that will continue to require consideration and resolution. Children do not always remain children; no doubt in due time donor conceived children as adults will be their own best advocates in pressing for greater openness about donors. A situation where legislation is introduced which reduces secrecy about donor insemination while maintaining donor anonymity creates contradictions which demand resolution. A closer look at the functions and consequences of donor anonymity is urgently required.

References

Barton, M., Walker, K. & Weisner, B. P. (1945). Artificial insemination. *British Medical Journal*, **1**, 130–4.

Blyth, E. (1990). Assisted reproduction: what's in it for children? *Children and Society*, **4**, 167–82.

Bowler, P. J. (1990). *Charles Darwin: The Man and His Influence*, pp. 250. London: Blackwell.

Bromham, D. R., Dalton, M. E. & Jackson, J. C. (eds.) (1990). *Philosophical Ethics in Reproductive Medicine*. pp. 261. Manchester University Press.

Bruce, N. (1990). On the importance of genetic knowledge. *Children and Society*, **4**, 183–96.

Daniels, K. R. (1988). Artifical insemination using donor semen and the issues of secrecy: the views of donors and recipient couples. *Social Science and Medicine*. **27**, 377–83.

Feversham Lord (Chairman) (1960) *Report of the Departmental Committee on Human Artificial Insemination*. Cmnd 1105. London: HMSO.

Gregoire, A. T. & Mayer, A. C. (1965). The impregnators. *Fertility and Sterility*. **16**, 130–4.

Haimes, E. (1988). Secrecy: what can artificial reproduction learn from adoption? *International Journal of Law and the Family*. **2**, 46–61.

McWhinnie, A. (1966). *Adopted Children: How They Grow Up*. London: Routledge and Kegan Paul.

Peel Sir J. (Chairman) (1973). Report of the Panel on Human Artificial Insemination. *British Medical Journal*. **2**, Suppl. Appendix V,3.

Russell, B. (1929). *Marriage and Morals*. pp. 254. New York: Loveright.

Snowden, R. & Mitchell, G. D. (1981). *The Artificial Family: A Consideration of Artificial Insemination by Donor*. pp. 138. London: Allen and Unwin.

Snowden, R., Mitchell, G. D. & Snowden, E. M. (1983) *Artificial Reproduction: A Social Investigation*. pp. 188. London: Allen and Unwin.

Thompson, W., Joyce, D. N. & Newton, J. R. (eds) (1984). *In-vitro Fertilisation and Donor Insemination*. pp. 355. London: RCOG.

Titmus, R. (1970). *The Gift Relationship*. pp. 339. London: Allen and Unwin.

Triselliotis, J. (1975). *In Search of Origins: The Experience of Adopted People*. pp. 177. Boston: Beacon.

Walby, C. & Symons, B. (1990). *Who Am I? Identity, Adoption and Human Fertilisation*. pp. 128. London: BAAF.

Warnock, M. (Chairperson) (1984) *Report of an Inquiry into Human Fertilisation and Embryology*. pp. 103. London: HMSO.

14

Developments in donor insemination and the law in the UK

I. D. COOKE

Introduction

The provision of a donor insemination service has changed dramatically in the last year or so in the United Kingdom. It is worth tracing the development of the processes that have shaped these changes. It is likely that similar evolution will occur elsewhere but it is important to understand the influences that have conspired to effect these events.

Following the publication of the Warnock Report in 1984 (HMSO) in which the philosophical issues that arose from the use of donor gametes were expanded, some time elapsed before such contentious issues were addressed by Government. During this time the Medical Research Council and the Royal College of Obstetricians and Gynaecologists combined forces to establish a Voluntary Licensing Authority (VLA) to encourage self-regulation by clinics and personnel involved in *in vitro* fertilization (IVF) and gamete intra-fallopian transfer (GIFT). The VLA established criteria for clinic functions and initiated site visits. It emphasized quality of service but allowed time for clinics to establish baseline data to demonstrate effective treatment regimes. It insisted on security of records and the use of local research ethical committees to approve changes in clinical practice. Research proposals were examined carefully from an ethical viewpoint. Most importantly it published an Annual Report collecting data from all units and showed that the range of outcomes varied directly with the size of the unit. It also developed ethical guidelines for the use of donor oocytes.

This body was on the whole an effective regulatory body but there were some problems with individual practitioners who chose to transfer excess numbers of embryos following IVF or oocytes at GIFT attracting much publicity and encouraging calls for stricter regulation. To make the point that it hoped that the Government would create a statutory licensing authority, the VLA changed its name to the interim licensing authority (ILA).

A Government White Paper was then published. It presented the elements of the Warnock Report that it considered could form the basis of future legislation and sought responses from interested parties. Following this consultation a second White Paper was published which gave the Government's view on what form the legislation should take and this again was circulated for consultation.

The Human Fertilization and Embryology Act

Subsequently the Human Fertilization and Embryology Bill was introduced into the House of Lords and became law in October 1990. There are a number of novel features relating to donor insemination (DI). The Human Fertilization and Embryology Authority was established to administer the Act and to be responsible for giving licences to operate treatment or storage services or to carry out research involving the use of gametes. Sperm could only be used or stored subject to the Act. Gametes must not, in general, be stored for longer than 10 years or embryos for more than 5 years.

A man married to a woman treated by DI becomes the legal father of the child as does the man who, although not married to the mother of the child, is her partner. The sperm donor is not to be treated as the father. Information about donors and persons to whom treatment services were provided is to be kept by the Authority. Specified information is to be made available (upon request and after counselling) at the age of 18 or under that age if the individual proposes to marry.

There were two further significant developments in social policy. The first was that the Act stipulated that all individuals treated must have received 'proper counselling'. The second was that, in deciding whether or not to treat a couple, the welfare of the future child had to be taken into account and, in particular, the child's need for a father.

During passage of the Bill the King's Fund was commissioned by the Department of Health to develop a framework for counselling. This led to the publication in January 1991 of 'Counselling for Regulated Infertility Treatments', the Report of the King's Fund Centre Counselling Committee. It addressed counselling needs relating to the provision of infertility services for treatment covered by the Act from which children are born following gamete donation who seek information about their origins. It examined the needs of all donors.

This report broke new ground in that it defined counselling, a task avoided in the Act. It identified counselling as having a number of components: information counselling, implications counselling, support counselling and lastly therapeutic counselling. Other issues discussed were the timing of this counselling and the financing of what would become a major component of this service. This led to consideration of the training of the counsellors, the establishing of training courses and monitoring of counselling services.

The three major components of a gamete donation service were discussed: the couple seeking treatment, the gamete donor and the resulting child. The content of counselling for each of these was listed and the need for supplementary written material identified.

The Human Fertilization and Embryology Authority was established by the Act. It set up Licensing and Information committees and one to devise the Code of Practice which would be the framework for implementing the Act. A Code of Practice draft document was prepared with an explanatory supplement and circulated for consultation for two months. The definitive Code of Practice was published on 1 August 1991; it made effective the legal basis for regulations for DI services and research. All clinics, storage and research facilities must be inspected within 12 months and licensed upon payment of the basic licence fee for registration depending on the activity: treatment, storage or research. In addition, unit charges are to be made for each cycle of DI treatment based initially on the previous year's statistics. To effect this, forms detailing each treatment cycle are to be returned to the Central Registry, a major increase in clerical work.

The Code of Practice

The Code of Practice provides details for all aspects of clinic functioning and regulations which empower the Authority to act in these areas.

Staff

One individual must be designated as 'the responsible person' who legally is responsible for all aspects of the operation of the clinic. A medical

practitioner experienced in infertility must have overall clinical responsibility for treatment services. A qualified registered nurse must be available in the clinic. Counselling staff must have formal qualifications or a
qualified counsellor must be available as adviser to staff and clients.
Formal academic or technical training and experience in semenology is
required for scientific staff. All staff require in-service training.

Facilities

Equipment and appropriate practices must be used. Comfort and privacy
both for patients and donors are emphasized and counselling must be
offered to all donors and recipients involved in storage, donation or
treatment. Access to outside counselling organizations must be made
available if appropriate. Secure storage of gametes is advised with
controlled access. Monitoring and evaluation of all aspects of the service
are required and feedback from all participants is encouraged. This
should lead to regular updating for all practices. Limits on advertising are
laid down.

Assessing clients, donors and the welfare of the child

The needs of the couple and those of the child are equally important and
both must be assessed before agreement to treatment is reached. Confidentiality has been taken to an extreme. Once it is intended to treat,
donate or store in a licensed centre any communication apart from that
with another licensed centre is illegal except through the patient him/
herself. All correspondence must be addressed to the patient and only
exact copies of the letters may be enclosed for the patient to forward to
the medical adviser, the referring doctor or another consultant where
advice is sought regarding the welfare of the treated person. Otherwise
on the consent form the exact wording must be specified before the
patient signs a release to send the letter direct to another doctor. These
restrictions have generated great administrative difficulties, created
resentment by referring practitioners and inhibited the traditional
exchange of medical detail. The lack of information available to those
caring for the patient outside the centre could create major problems in
an emergency. It seems likely that this unintended and cumbersome
restriction will be modified at the first opportunity.*

---

* This confidentiality provision was relaxed on a 'need to know' basis in recent supple-
mentry legislation.

The prospective parents must be evaluated as potential parents within their family structure. There are aspects such as commitment to bringing up a child, their ages, and medical histories, the prospects of multiple birth, risks to the child(ren) and the impact on other members of the family. Great emphasis is placed on the child's potential need to know about his or her origins and whether or not the prospective parents can cope with a child's questions when growing up. The attitude of other family members and the implications for the child should be taken into account.

Particular emphasis is placed upon recognizing a support structure if the female to be inseminated is unsupported. Parental preferences in physical characteristic matching should be acknowledged. Background enquiries from the general practitioner or another agency are encouraged if they throw light on the potential social risks of the treatment. The patient's consent for the seeking of this information must be given but refusal could be interpreted as a reason for denying treatment. The assessment of a couple is recognized as being multidisciplinary and this could lead to refusal to provide treatment, but an explanation for reasons for such a decision should be given, further options explained and access to relevant counselling offered. The reasons for all these decisions should be recorded.

Prospective donors and those seeking gamete storage should all be counselled and then screened for human immunodeficiency virus (HIV). Payment for donations is defined in regulations which limit the sum and foreshadow abolition in two years. There appears to be enthusiasm for a genuine donation without payment of all semen samples as practised by CECOS in France since 1973 (CECOS Report, 1991). However, the prospect of seeing or screening adequate numbers of donors in the UK where payment is being practised routinely may be more difficult without payment.

Male donors should not usually be older than 55 years nor under 18. Sperm may be taken from younger males for their own later treatment or with their valid consent for research. The history should be ascertained and enquiry made of general practitioners for background in those offering to be donors or requiring storage of their gametes.

In addition to the above screening, the potential fertility of the sample, whether or not the donor has children and the attitude of the donor to donation should be taken into account. Infection screening and rescreening are recommended. Rejection of a donor for any reason should be explained and relevant counselling offered.

Information

Both oral and written information must be given by suitably trained individuals to all clients for treatment, donation or storage. Details of outcome of treatment, logistics, methods, cost, limitations and length of treatment should be given. The recipients need to know about counselling and that the welfare of the child will be taken into account in making treatment decisions. They need to know about central registration of data. They must understand the child's potential need to know about its origins and its right to seek that information in due course. Recognition of who will become the designated parents is required, particularly in treatment of couples from abroad.

Donors need to know about methods of gamete collection, HIV screening and quarantine. They should understand that their anonymity is protected under the Act, that only non-identifying information can be released subsequently to the child and that they will not be regarded as a parent of any child born. There is normally to be a limit of ten children born to any one donor unless a lower number is specified by the donor.

The donor needs to know the purpose to which the donation may be put and that any congenital anomaly arising as a result of his failure to disclose defects about which he knew or ought reasonably to have known may allow him to be sued for damages.

Consent

Forms for consent to treatment in general have recently been revised by the Department of Health but the Code of Practice provides a new form for consent to DI treatment. A suitable time for reflection by the patient after receiving information should be allowed to elapse before the consent is obtained.

Consent should also be obtained if there are to be any observers during treatment procedures.

A woman's husband would be the legal father of any child conceived although his written consent should be obtained. If he does not consent, a written statement to that effect should be obtained. A male partner could similarly be regarded as the father of the child and that should be explained and the partner's attendance at each clinic visit recorded. A donor should consent in writing to the maximum period of storage, normally 10 years. A more prolonged scale is allowable if storage is required for personal use, for example after treatment of a malignancy when the duration is greater the younger the person.

The donor should state what should happen to his gametes if he dies or becomes incapable of varying or revoking his consent. He should consent to their use for treatment including the creation of an embryo. If the embryo is to be created *in vitro*, the purpose must be stated, for treatment or research. There should be time for reflection before consent is signed, and the donor should not feel under pressure.

Counselling

The concepts of counselling already formulated by the King's Fund Committee have been used in the Code of Practice. Information, the professional clinical relationship, and the process of assessment prior to accepting a donor are emphatically distinguished from other counselling which is offered as optional. The implications of the proposed treatment or donation must be explored. However, support for stress experienced in the face of failure to achieve a pregnancy, or therapeutic counselling, for the causes or consequences of the infertility treatment (which may be directed at acceptance of the situation) are optional.

Counselling should be part of the routine service and determined by the patient's need. It should be seen as separate from routine clinical management and should be available to individuals or couples. The opportunity for counselling should arise after the initial oral or written information has been given and digested. There are many implications to be considered: the responsibility of the centre in ensuring a good outcome, of its impact on themselves, family, social circle and any resulting child; what are the pros and cons of being open about the treatment and explaining it to relatives and friends? Couples should consider their attitude to their own or their partner's infertility and the potential of failed treatment. They should consider feelings about not being the genetic father of the child, how they perceive the child's needs throughout growth and development and how these feelings may change with time. Donors should consider the use and possible disposal of any embryos derived from their gametes. Whenever a woman is undergoing IVF and a failed fertilization arises or its possibility is envisaged, counselling for the use of donated gametes should take place separately from the treatment and before it begins.

Counselling of donors should cover their reasons for wanting to be donors, their attitudes to any resulting children and their willingness to forego knowledge and responsibility for such children. They should consider the needs of those children and their own attitudes to the legal parents of these children. The issue of their own possible future infertility should be raised. Their attitudes to research on embryos derived from their gametes should be ascertained. A partner of a potential donor should also be offered counselling.

Counselling may be requested either during or after donation or treatment and should also be countenanced. Persons for whom treatment has failed or who have refused treatment, and donors who have declined or had unsuspected defects identified may require support counselling or access to an infertility support group. Centre staff should be trained to be aware of the need for, and provide, such support. Therapeutic counselling may be required for problems that may, or may not, be associated with the infertility and access to such help should be arranged. Finally, a record should be made of all counselling offered, and whether it was accepted or not.

Use of gametes (and embryos)

Transport of sperm is only permitted between licensed centres or according to directions allowing import or export. Care should be exercised that the development potential of gametes is not being harmed in any way and that no contamination has occurred. Women should be treated in any one cycle with the gametes of only one man. Only in exceptional situations should more than ten live children be born from any one donor.

Storage and handling of gametes

Controlled access to secure areas where gametes are stored is only allowed to named individuals. All gamete handling and location should be monitored and recorded in detail. Gamete source and subsequent fate should be traceable at all times and regular reviews should take place. Transfer of gametes should be carefully undertaken.

Research

All projects should be licensed separately. The only subject areas in which projects relating to sperm will be licensed are those to promote advances in the treatment of infertility, to increase knowledge of the causes of congenital disease or miscarriages or to develop more effective techniques of contraception. All proposals must first be reviewed by an Ethics Committee. Gametes which are being used for research cannot subsequently be used for treatment.

Records

A named individual should be responsible for all records and related transactions. Access by donors and patients to information about themselves should be allowed.

Complaints

A complaints procedure should be established and notices of the procedure displayed. Assistance in formulating a complaint should be given if required and then investigation should follow with the outcome being reported to the complainant. Notification of the number of complaints should be made annually to the Authority.

Comment

The above detailed presentation of the contents of the Code of Practice provides a framework for all work involving DI in the United Kingdom. It and IVF are the only two medical treatment procedures subject to sanctions under the criminal law. Regular inspections to appraise quality control will be undertaken by the regulatory Authority which will collect and publish the statistical returns including the outcome of pregnancies which centres are required to notify.

Although Sweden has legislated to remove the cloak of anonymity from semen donors, no other country has laid down such rigorous controls which are subject to a legal framework and inspection. In March, 1990, the American Fertility Society (AFS) published its new guidelines for use of donor insemination which were recommendations for good practice. More specific recommendations were made, for example, relating to infection screening which are not defined in the UK Code. Appendices cover selection and screening of donors and minimal genetic screening for the donors.

In June 1990, the Ethics Committee of the AFS published Ethical Considerations of the New Reproductive Technologies. Included in the discussion of DI was the view that 'in order to avoid the problems of inappropriate motivation . . . no payment should be made for the semen donation although compensation for time and expenses incurred by the donor is acceptable'.

The next year will see the impact of these new regulations on DI practice in the UK. Already a number of clinics have closed presumably because of real or imagined difficulties in complying with the stringent Code of Practice or because of the considerable charges to be levied by the Authority. Doubtless standards and in-service provision will rise but hopefully not at the expense of a gross reduction in the availability to the population. Development of counselling will proceed from an uncertain base but the resources both human and economic to fulfil the ideal provision may be long in coming. It is to be hoped that the legal entanglement and the increased difficulty of working and communicating created by this legisation will not militate against easier access by those in need. If a long-term effect is to escalate costs beyond the means of the average person, the achievement of high standards will have been a Pyrrhic victory.

References

Warnock Report (1984). HMSO.
Code of Practice (1991). Human Fertilization and Embryology Authority, Clements House, 14–18 Gresham Street, London EC2V 7JE.
Human Fertilization and Embryology Act (1990).
Counselling for Regulated Infertility Treatments (1991). King's Fund Centre.
The Sixth Report of the Interim Licensing Authority for Human *in vitro* Fertilization and Embryology (1991). ILA.
New guidelines for the use of semen donor insemination (1990). *Fertility and Sterility*, **53**, Suppl. 1.
Ethical considerations of the new reproductive technologies, *Fertility and Sterility*, **53**, Suppl. 2.

15

Computerization of a Donor Insemination Unit

H. LEACH and I. C. MACLEOD

Since the Donor Insemination service was instituted, it has grown considerably in size and complexity. Thus, the quantity of paperwork, data and information handling and the need for accurate statistical reports has grown accordingly.

The solution to the problem of a growing management workload, with little room for error, may be overcome by employing more staff. However, economic aspects apart, this can never be the ideal strategy to adopt since the function of a DI unit is best served by a small administrative team. Increases in staffing generate more management planning, communication and procedures. There is a greater likelihood of conflict and failure of human performance.

Organizations have developed and used electronic data processing systems since the mid-1960s. Such systems, using mainframe hardware and in-house programmers, prohibit all but the large organizations on the basis of economies of scale.

The introduction of computer mini/micro systems, in the early 1980s, allowed small organizations in particular, to take advantage of such systems as a way of obtaining greater efficiency in their operation. Only recently, however, have the appropriate software processing techniques been developed to cope with precise requirements in an efficient manner and within budget constraints, a leading example is the use of relational databases with built-in application generators, which allow users to customize the existing database package to the individual needs of the system (dBase IV, Aickin (1989), Richardson *et al.*, 1990).

Developments within information technology have produced many good database software packages. However, these packages need to be

214

far more than a standard database. They should be user friendly, up to date, and a day-by-day working data management instrument. In this sense, the customization process is evident. Thus computerized operations using the database will perform tasks that would otherwise be prohibitive.

Before any such system can be developed, it must be thoroughly analysed and designed to fit user requirements, using up to date methodologies. There are various development techniques and lifestyle models on which to build systems upon, e.g. SSADM (structured systems analysis and design methodology (Cutts, 1987)), JSP (Jackson structures programming) or the Yourdon SSAM (structured systems analysis methodology).

Design of a new system suggests that it is not a question of direct conversion of existing procedures and practices. It provides an ideal point in time to re-evaluate the existing system and take advantage of the benefits computerization can offer. Manual systems allow access only by the index in which they are stored, any relating information needing to be extracted and analysed must be carried out manually. A computer can enable multiple indexes to be created, linked files and access to complicated sorting on almost any relative field or multiple indexed fields (Jones, 1988a,b). Computer information/data is stored once but the output may take many different forms. For example, a patient's name and address can be used on invoices, their medical records, letters and appointments. The donor can be linked with his semen analysis report, the number of donations made, the calculations of payment to donors, his medical test results and numbers of pregnancies resulting.

The aim of such a program should be to simplify the day-to-day operation for the users. Therefore, the first step when planning such a programme is to determine what features the operational system contains.

If the program were used by a single user for record keeping and appointment generating a straightforward specification of the outputs would be listed for the program to generate. A multiuser program, on the other hand, perhaps run as a networked system, may offer more complex operations such as financial analysis, accounts, report generation and complex sorting. A complex analysis of the program specification would be required.

The analysis of a large system would require a systems analyst, having the benefit of a software engineering approach based on structured standards and agreed procedures. There will be need to carry out a complete study of the organization for which the program is being written, including collecting written materials and reports already in use, interviewing users, design and creation of data flow diagrams to show the data network and what changes are made on the way. Presentations of the findings at strategic stages of the analysis and design are necessary to keep the users up to date regarding developments and to confirm that the analysis is correct up to that particular stage (structured systems analysis and design methodology).

The result of the analysis should contain a list of all the required tasks within the program, together with the input and output options of the user, screen designs and form layouts (Cutts, 1987).

During the initial stages, consideration should be made as to the precise nature of the information to be stored, and registration under the Data Protection Act, 1987 may be necessary. The decision must be made regarding access by patients and donors to the information stored relating directly to them (The Data Protection Act, 1985).

For security and privacy reasons there must be access levels placed on the data so that users have limited access to those parts of the program which relate only to the work that they do. Also the donor must not be easily identified at any stage or time by unauthorized users manipulating the related stored data.

Report screens are one of the greatest sources of information to the user, but are less likely to be presented to accountants, or shown off to other centres within a similar working environment, at conferences, seminars, etc. Designing the reports or end results is an ideal start when designing the new system. Once an agreement has been achieved regarding what the system is to produce, it can be written around these report layouts using a commercial Database package, e.g. dBase IV (Jones, 1988c).

Screens should be planned with careful consideration of the officer who will enter the data. They would appreciate having to move the cursor in one direction when entering a new field of information. Consider the forms as point of generation for the data, and in what order this needs to be entered.

When converting the existing manual process to a computerized system, the following facilities will be required:

1. Enquiry programs to enable on screen enquiries.
2. Transaction programs to post data to different files.
3. Report programs, designed to give a hard copy of data.

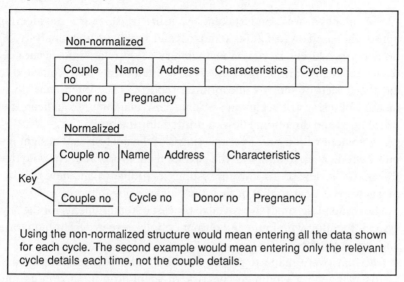

Fig. 15.1. Normalized and non-normalized file structures.

4. Batch routines to enable backups of the system.
5. A menu program which will link all these elements together.
6. Any special program functions that will produce calculations and complex queries.

The analysis of the system should have provided the developer with a file structure or what is termed a data dictionary. This is simply a list of all entities and the attributes associated with each one. The files should be normalized before defining within the computer program. This means deciding on a key for each file and a linked key for joining files, thus enabling data to be stored once only, yet used within several reports and screen layouts (Fig. 15.1).

Each file structure carries the same amount of information but the normalized file has data stored once only. Repeated data is stored in separate files as transactions. This is advisable as data which occurs more than once may miss being updated in one or more parts of the program, or be mistakenly updated more than once. Note that data can be read and displayed in almost any format so it is best not to use screen displays or reports as file structures.

At the Infertility Research Trust in Sheffield, a computerized system has been developing over the past two years, to cater for the growing demands upon the existing manual system for semen analysis and donor insemination.

The analysis was undertaken by using a software engineering approach, based on structures standards and agreed systems analysis and design procedures. It was vital to interview all staff and accurately document their working processes. All printed forms were collected to aid the design of screens and printed reports. The system was documented by using the technique of data flow diagrams, to indicate the procedures and directional flow of printed documents.

Agreement with users at various stages of the analysis and design, not only kept them up to date with the development process but checked that the analyst's view of the current system, its problems and new requirements were as near to that of the user's view as possible.

The result of the analysis proved to be a list of requirements for the new system, together with input and output options, screen designs and form and report layouts.

Decisions were made regarding security and access levels and passwords planned to eliminate the risk of identification of donors and couples by unauthorized personnel.

The main objectives within the development were to allow the following.

1. Data collection and storage on a daily basis from all areas within the DI service, i.e. nurses, clinicians, technicians and scientists.
2. Donor selection, assisting the clinician by providing a list of suitable donors for a particular patient, selecting on specified criteria, e.g. blood group, hair, eye and skin colouring.
3. Financial analysis, providing a stock control facility, and an accounting module to record expenses paid to donors, payments received from couples for treatment, and payment from other clinics for semen sold.
4. Statistical analysis, from which data could easily be transferred to other packages for statistical analysis and accurate pregnancy per donor records in accordance with the legislation specified by the Human Fertilization and Embryology Authority (HFEA, 1991).

Hardware

The unit had a small ethernet local area network installed, which comprised 4 IBM compatible PCs. The network had been used previously to run a commercially available database package for simple storage and retrieval of data.

Since the present hardware was to be used, it was felt best to upgrade the fileserver to a PC with a faster processor and larger hard disk capacity to allow housing for the main DI program; statistics packages and the unit accounts software would be linked at a later stage to the DI software.

The remaining 3 PCs were used as workstations. Each had a 40 mb hard drive and were to be used as stand alone PCs when not in use for the DI program; these required no modification. The workstations were positioned to allow for data entry as near as possible to the data generation, i.e. clinic, lab office and DI office.

Software

It was decided to develop the software using a commercially available fourth generation language package which offered powerful relational database features based on a data dictionary format. Once the code was generated and compiled, the program would run on any IBM compatible PC running MSDOS. Single or multiuser versions could be generated, and any modifications easily maintained by changing the structure of the module and re-generating. The program structure was modular to allow for expansion as necessary. An example would be to add extra reports, data entry screens, etc.

Since nurses, technicians, clinicians, counsellors and scientists were to operate various parts of the program, no prior knowledge of computer applications was assumed. It was therefore thought best to develop a program which was menu driven. Passwords and user levels were agreed, allowing access to a limited set of menu options, as the password and user level dictated.

A password entry to the system from each terminal was initiated upon turning on the computer and allowed access only to the programs stored on the terminal's hard drive. Failure to enter the correct password after three attempts would result in the system aborting and the hard disc being locked. Re-setting the machine presented the prompt to enter the password once again. A further password and user level codes had to be entered upon entry to the DI program, stored on the hard drive of the fileserver, thus setting the access levels to the menu screens.

Problems encountered throughout development

From the analysis stage it was obvious that the main difficulty would be to overcome the resistance to change, demonstrated by some members of staff. At the time of development, there was little computer awareness within the department, and a certain amount of uncertainty and distrust regarding the accuracy of computer-generated reports.

A series of simple training sessions were arranged to help develop computer awareness, and to ease the fears of computer shy staff. The training sessions also helped to demonstrate that if data is entered incorrectly, accurate reports cannot be produced (GIGO, garbage in, garbage out).

Once staff began to feel more familiar with using the computer as a technical tool, they began to come to terms with the changing role of computerization within the department.

There were also those who were under the impression that computerization would remove a huge amount of routine work within the department, when, in fact, some jobs were actually duplicated, e.g. treatment data, after being recorded in patient records at the time of treating, needed entry into the computer afterwards. Similarly, information regarding donor semen analyses would be recorded on a form to be later transcribed into the computer system.

Data processing was the main advantage of the computerized system; however, manual records still had to be maintained. At a later stage, some manual records may be taken over completely by electronic data stores, but it was felt best to run the two systems concurrently until the computer system could take over completely.

Security of data

Security of the data was of utmost importance and the need for a reliable form of back-up necessary.

A tape streamer was purchased to increase data security and reduce the time spent in backing up the system with floppy discs. It was far more reliable and one tape holds 120 mb of data. The whole of the network could be successfully backed up in less than 30 minutes and a single file deleted inadvertently could be replaced within minutes.

Compatibility and co-ordination with other software

Data is stored in a format which is directly compatible with commercially available software packages, and can be easily transferred into most recognized database, spreadsheet, wordprocessing and statistical analysis packages which not only run on IBM compatible PCs but on the large mainframe system housed in the main University Computing Department. It is hoped at a later stage of development to include files, taken directly from the Department's Hamilton Thorn Motility analyser within parts of the DI program.

Conclusions

Computerization of the administrative and research procedures within the unit is a classic example of a system which incorporates routines that could not be performed by manual methods. Therefore, in summary, a computerized system exhibits the following characteristics.

1. The ability to handle a wide range of variables, where outputs are produced within the database.
2. High-speed execution with efficient and error-free results.
3. Historic reporting, which complements current and future research.
4. Consistency in the context of changing staff, both administrative and technical, together with permanent and temporary research staff.
5. Provision of an initial reference datum and for a range of outputs within changing constraints but leaving room for expansion of alternative strategies.

One extremely valuable advantage of such a program is that it can be easily arranged and analysed to answer basic scientific questions, for example, the influence of female age on fecundability. Life table analysis, involving sophisticated tabled tests, e.g. Cox's regression model (see chapter 12) can easily be implemented.

Notwithstanding the advantage of such a system, the efficiency of outputs and reports is relative to the accuracy of data input verification. Input by the best operatives would not be 100%, therefore a periodic audit is essential to allow certification and guaranteed authenticity. A continuous training program within the unit would be necessary with stringent specifications to ensure the high standards necessary in this field.

References

Aickin, M. (1989). A simple dBase programme for medical studies. *Computing Methods Programs*, Biomed [DOH] **28**, 201–5.
Cutts, G. (1987). *Structures, Systems Analysis and Design Methodology*. Blackwell. 425.
The Data Protection Registrar (1985). The Data Protection Act 1984.

Human Fertilization and Embryology Authority (1991). Code of Practice. Clements House, 14–18 Gresham Street, London EC2V 7JE.

Jones, E. (1988a). *Relational Databases from Using dBase IV*, p. 9, USA: Osborne McGraw-Hill.

Jones, E. (1988b). *Database Design, from Using dBase IV*, pp. 18–25, USA: Osborne McGraw-Hill.

Jones, E. (1988c). *Using the Applications Generator, from Using dBase IV*, pp. 437–67, USA: Osborne McGraw-Hill.

Richardson, C. A., Dickinson, A. S., Barratt, C. L. R. & Cooke, I. D. (1990). Using a donor insemination management system. *British Medical Bulletin* **46**, 813–22.

16
Concluding remarks

I. D. COOKE

This book has comprehensively outlined DI: management of patients, guidelines for DI, success rates and how to calculate them and ethical and legal aspects have been considered. Many points are worthy of further discussion. However, for convenience four principal areas will be discussed.

Donors

It is clear that the difficulties of screening and selecting donors, particularly in the United Kingdom with the new HFEA legislation, have led to acute problems in recruiting sufficient numbers. CECOS (who have the most comprehensive database in the world) have a system which does not involve rigorous screening of the donor prior to donation as in America and the UK. The number of congenital abnormalities in DI children is not increased in the CECOS system compared to the general population, so the CECOS protocol would appear appropriate. It is important to remember that CECOS only recruit donors who already have children and are in stable relationships. This is not so in the United Kingdom and the United States where the donor base is young people who have often not had children. In the UK there will be pressure to change in the near future, and the experience of the CECOS system is likely to be a valuable guide for many centres.

There is a distinct need to improve the examination of the fertilizing capacity of semen so that only high quality semen is used in the donor insemination system. Appropriate sperm function tests, e.g. the measurement of reactive oxygen species and quantitative motility should be performed prior to a donor being accepted onto a programme. It is probable that only a few centres will be able to perform these tests, and perhaps these centres could supply other centres with semen of very high quality. This would represent a major challenge to centres in the United Kingdom. A system does operate in CECOS, although the sperm function testing of the donors is not as sophisticated.

There is a clear need to improve the cryopreservation of donor semen. The use of various media and freeze/thaw protocols clearly require rigorous scientific testing with clear biological end points.

Female partners

One of the major barriers to success in donor insemination is the fecundity of the female. Clearly such factors as ovulatory defects and damaged tubes compromise conception. However, there is still controversy over other more 'minor' problems, e.g. endometriosis. There is still also controversy over the degree of investigation prior to treatment. There is an argument that only a minimum investigation apart from detection of ovulation should be performed. If a pregnancy does not occur, after a certain number of cycles the female should be investigated. This may be reasonable if the husband is azoospermic, but, if sperm are present in the semen, the chances of success in DI are significantly lower and therefore the female should be investigated. This does, however, depend on the waiting for investigations which may be excessive. The role of superovulation as an empirical treatment with DI still remains to be established. Timing of ovulation using accurate techniques is now available, yet prospective randomized trials need to be performed to ascertain the value of these measurements. If sperm are present in the male partner prior to donor insemination, their function needs to be addressed. This can be done using appropriate sperm function testing, so as to determine which men have potentially fertile spermatozoa and may be better off having an homologous test fertilization at IVF. The question of when couples should be referred for GIFT or IVF is also a matter of controversy and would undoubtedly depend on the cost effectiveness and efficiency of each system.

Research

The donor insemination system can be used in research to answer biological questions. In addressing many of these questions, accurate computerized databases and appropriate statistical techniques are mandatory and will aid data analysis. The inadequate use of statistics in reproductive medicine has been widely critized in the literature. Life table analysis and Cox's regression, however, are ideal for use in donor insemination to identify which factors influence success. They can also be used to help in the design of prospective trials. Clinical management of the patients will also be helped by the availability of this data, e.g. providing instant data on the number of pregnancies per donor, the number of donors in stock, the number of donors needing to be recruited over the next 6 months, the number of patients awaiting treatment, etc.

Counselling

Changes in recent UK law have made counselling mandatory for couples having DI. There are insufficient trained counsellors available for this to happen immediately; mechanisms for training and the unique skill of counselling and experience of management of infertility needs to be defined. It is now stated that a child has a right to know his/her origins by DI and more details of the donor. Long term follow-up must establish the validity of this assertion for DI and assess the impact on the child, family and on the donor. Extensive counselling of couples now prepares them better for DI, and society at large is more aware of the problems and treatment. Nevertheless, the way in which couples who attempt to be open about their DI are received by other people will need to be carefully monitored and interpreted. It will be of particular interest to see how many offspring of DI request further information from the Registry of the HFEA when they reach 16–18 years of age.

In summary, there have been advances in donor insemination which have been clearly outlined. However, many questions still remain to be answered. It is hoped that this book will stimulate research to ask appropriate biological questions in donor insemination. It is important, also, to recognize that donor insemination will not only be used in the clinical management of men with male infertility, but also in the future will be used for single women and men who are HIV positive where the female is negative. Donor insemination provides a challenging reproductive technology for the future.

Index

RG
134
D63